The book describes a series of programmatic solutions that make medical care more readily available. None of them are firmly institutionalized. They may survive budget constraints and become permanent parts of the complex of access services or they may disappear from the health care scene. In any case, they represent important initiatives necessary if hospital-based health care services are to be more effective, and in the patient's interest.

Helen Rehr, who has recently retired as Director of the Department of Social Work Services at the Mount Sinai Hospital, continues as Special Assistant to the Executive Vice President, representing the hospital in its work with the community. Within the Mount Sinai School of Medicine, she is the Edith J. Baerwald Professor of Community Medicine (Social Work), Director of the Division of Social Work Continuing Education, Director of the Murray M. Rosenberg Applied Social Work Research Center and Co-principal Investigator of the Brookdale Social-Health Center for the Aging. She also holds a Clinical Professorship at the Brookdale Center for the Aging at Hunter College, as well as Adjunct Professor at the Hunter College School of Social Work, and has served in a number of visiting professorships including the Kenneth L. Pray post at the University of Pennsylvania. She has written extensively for professional journals and has brought out several books on health-oriented social work practice, the most recent of which is *Professional Accountability for Social Work*. She has been honored by admission to the Hunter College Hall of Fame, and as a recipient of the Ida M. Cannon Award for the Society for Hospital Social Work Directors of the American Hospital Association.

Mildred D. Mailick is an Associate Professor at Hunter College School of Social Work, City University of New York, where she coordinates the Social Health Concentration. She has written extensively for professional journals and lectured in professional forums on social work practice, advocacy and interprofessional collaboration in h
tings. Dr. Mailick is an ex
representative and ombuds
and has served as a consult
pitals in the United Sta
countries.

D0929837

In the Patient's Interest:
ACCESS TO HOSPITAL CARE

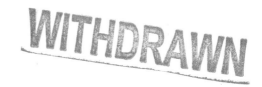

In the Patient's Interest

Access to Hospital Care

Edited by
Mildred D. Mailick
Helen Rehr

PRODIST
New York 1981

Published in the United States by
PRODIST, a division of
Neale Watson Academic Publications, Inc.
156 Fifth Avenue, New York, N.Y. 10010

Library of Congress Catologing in Publication Data

Main entry under title:

In the patient's interest.

   1. Hospital and community. 2. Hospital care.
3. Hospital patients. 4. Hospital care—United States.
I. Mailick, Mildred. II. Rehr, Helen. [DNLM: 1. Health
services accessibility—United States. 2. Hospitals—
United States. 3. Patient advocacy. WX 27 AA1 I35]
RA965.5.I5   362.1'1   81–15781
ISBN 0–88202–136–2   AACR2

Designed and manufactured in the U.S.A.

Tributes

We wish to pay tribute to the memory of two persons who assisted in the realization of this book. The first is Helen Haberman Deitch, who as a full-time volunteer at The Mount Sinai Hospital loved her work as a patient representative. Her past successful experiences in business and in advertising were translated quickly to health care delivery. She brought with her an interest in medical matters and an interest in people. These skills made her a natural advocate for others, and *In The Patient's Interest* is a fulfillment of that commitment to advocacy. She contributed a chapter to this book, but it was her warm support of us in the continuance of the project which was her most cherished contribution. While she did not live to see its publication, she saw the manuscript and assisted in the review of it.

The second tribute is to Philip W. Haberman, Jr. It was Helen's wish that the Philip W. Haberman, Jr. Fund should support the original research in patient representatives and it did so generously.

This book is dedicated, as Helen Haberman Deitch wrote it:
"In memory of Philip W. Haberman, Jr.,
Trustee of The Mount Sinai Hospital, 1938–1971"

Contents

Acknowledgments

Many people were important in helping this book to reach publication. First, we wish to express special appreciation to the Auxiliary Board of The Mount Sinai Hospital, first with Mrs. Seymour M. Klein, followed by Mrs. Stephen L. Wolf during their terms as President, for their ongoing interest and guidance, and for the Board's financial support in sponsoring the publication of *In The Patient's Interest.* Ruth Ravich, a pioneer patient representative, gave counsel, graciously shared her knowledge and experience, and provided access to important early patient representative documents. Thanks are also due to Arline Sax and Alix Gekas of the Society of Patient Representatives of the American Hospital Association who assisted in the data gathering. There were twenty-eight health care professionals in seven hospitals, who, although they remain anonymous, contributed generously in their interviews about their experiences with patient representative programs. Their responses added authenticity to the study and we are especially grateful to them for their openness and for their candor. Margery Levenstein was helpful in reading for continuity and then in typing the manuscript. Suzanne Rauffenbart offered wise consultation. Finally, we wish to thank Dorothy Nayer who edited the manuscript with knowledge and care.

Preface

A unique characteristic of the health care industry is that the providers of hospital services do not market the product directly to the consumer. Instead, the physician serves as the intermediary, and the patient becomes the end user of the product at the physician's direction.

A patient actually receives two types of services in a hospital: the "professional" services—the diagnostic tests, surgery and other forms of treatment and the "patient caring" services—reflected in the attitudes of all staff and in the quality of the "hotel" type functions—housekeeping, food service, billing, etc. Most patients do not have sufficient expertise to judge the "professional" services they receive so they very frequently form their opinion of the hospital on the quality of the "caring" services.

This consumer phenomenon places great importance on the role of the patient representative who provides a support system for the patient and identifies services which are not satisfying patient needs.

As hospitals move into a more competitive environment in the 1980's, management must take a closer look at data collected by patient representatives and on other forms of consumer opinion of hospital services.

We need to know what consumers think about us. Just as private industries do market surveys of the people who use their services, hospitals must develop useful data on how patient services are received and perceived by the consumer. This book provides an introduction to the patient perspective of hospital services. Its message is a vital one for all health professionals. Each of us—administrators, nurses, social workers, therapists, and physicians—must more carefully evaluate our services from the patient perspective. We must create an environment in which the patients perceive that their needs are being met. The authors have set the stage for us. We now must do it.

Samuel Davis, Director, The Mount Sinai Hospital

Introduction

The health care system in the United States reflects in microcosm many of the problems of the society as a whole. Health services have become more complex, more highly technical, specialized, fragmented, and difficult to reach. Access to services is inequitably affected by economic, social, and racial considerations. The system is multifaceted, consisting of a patchwork of private entrepreneurial practitioners and proprietary, voluntary, and public institutions. Planning can be fragmented and erratic, frequently shaped by the personal decision-making of individual professionals, powerful medical and hospital associations, and local, state, and federal bodies.

Individual choice is constricted by a myriad of mechanistic regulations, lack of information about rights, benefits, and resources. Barriers to health care are also sometimes self-erected by personal predilections, biases, cultural patterns, and life styles. Yet with all of this, personal expectations for health and health care are rising. There is a growing demand for access to individualized, humane, and comprehensive health services.

This book is concerned with access to hospital-based health care services. The focus is on hospitals alone, since they are the major cost center of all the health services. Hospitals are a key factor in the organization of the health care system. There has been a shift in the locus of service from the medical bag of old-fashioned general practitioners to the laboratories and treatment facilities of large hospitals. Physicians tend to cluster around hospitals so they can draw on supportive resources: consultants, technicians, nurses, hospital beds, and machines. Hospital costs constitute the largest single expenditure of the health care dollar, and control of access to hospitals has great implications for the cost of medical care. More and more of the general public are using hospital facilities for primary medical care. Patients who may need other forms of care find themselves inappropriately in hospital beds and use emergency rooms and outpatient clinics when they neither wish them nor can afford them. Once themselves inappropriately in hospital beds and use emergency rooms and outpatient clinics when they neither wish them nor can afford them. Once in hospitals, they then encounter obstacles to ongoing care. Thus, helping people gain entry to appropriate hospital services and using the facilities soundly is in every patient's interest.

Part One focuses on the breakdown in access to health services. Chapter One considers the issues and problems raised by existing access patterns to medical institutions. It identifies access as the critical factor in the health care system, defining who gets service, how it is provided, and how followed up. Using the concept of barriers to access, it assesses obstacles to services in two major systems: provider and consumer. It sees the interaction between these two systems as complex, encompassing social, environmental, economic, cultural, psychological, and organizational influences.

The hospital as the focal point of the health care system is assessed in the second chapter. Some of the kaleidoscopic changes in the health care scene are noted. The implications of these changes for patients seeking services are identified. The focus is on patients rather than on institutions or providers. Patients seeking services are seen as the least powerful of the interacting forces, needing the most assistance in overcoming barriers to service.

Advocacy on behalf of the consumer group is receiving increasing attention in health care delivery. Many dynamic new programs are being developed and old programs are being strengthened. All have potential for improving the interaction between consumer and provider. The editors have selected a number of the most promising mechanisms of patient advocacy that seem especially pertinent to the construct of access as here defined. Information and referral services and community-based ombudsman programs are described as the new programs which assist patients to cross the threshold of hospitals and, in some cases, to return to the community. Patient representative programs are one major innovative approach to assist patients once inside hospital doorways to continue to find and use appropriate services within the institution. The focus on these three types of programs, which deal with overcoming obstacles to service, represents a major approach to the idea of opening up access.

In Part Two, community-based programs are examined. Information and referral services discussed in Chapter Three are a rapidly expanding form of service linking the consumer in need to all kinds of appropriate resources. The application of this type of service to the health field has considerable potential. It provides help to individuals in defining problems and identifying services available to alleviate them. It increases the consumer's potential choices by providing up-to-date information about resources. It refers consumers to acceptable facilities and follows through to ensure that the service is satisfactory. It helps to improve services for patients by identifying gaps and insufficiencies in the health care system and feeding these back to hospitals and other health care planning agencies. The community health ombudsman programs, described in Chapter Four, constitute a different approach to patient advocacy. While all ombudsmen programs provide information about institutional programs and thus increase access, some of them have as their major role the monitoring of the quality of care being received by patients. Programs vary in the degree to which they take on an adversary role with the providers of care. Most make some attempt at identifying injustices on the basis of investigation of patient complaints and suggest changes in policy and program.

Part Three looks at a major new form of patient advocacy within the hospital. Patient representative programs have grown in number in a remarkably short period of time. Like all new dynamic programs they are somewhat controversial. Chapter Five describes the patient representative program, the forces encouraging its development, and the functions it performs in hospitals. Chapter Six discusses early studies of patient representative programs and then presents in detail seven case studies of the development of different types of patient representative programs. Chapter Seven continues to exploit the case study method to explore how professionals—administrators, social work directors, nursing directors, and patient representatives—view the newly developing programs. These professionals present both advocate and adversary opinions about the patient representative programs, providing the reader, especially those who must work closely with the newly developed service, with some interesting perspectives.

In Part Four, which deals with conclusions, a retrospective and prospective view of access is presented. Chapter Eight gives a brief history of the Society of Patient Representatives and describes its purposes. In Chapter Nine, the editors broaden the scope of the problem of access and deal with it more comprehensively by making recommendations to deal with obstacles to services needed by consumers. While many programs are suggested, particular emphasis is placed on three innovative systems: information and referral, community based advocacy and patient representative.

The purpose of this book is thus to set out for the reader's inspection a series of possible programmatic solutions. None of them are firmly institutionalized. They may survive budget constraints and become permanent parts of the complex of access services or they may disappear from the health care scene. In any case, they represent attempts to find ways to respond more effectively in patients' interests.

Part I.

Access to Hospitals

Chapter I

Access to Services:
A Complex Dimension

HELEN REHR

Access is the single most critical factor in securing health care. It is a complex dynamic that involves prospective users and providers, as well as a range of sociopolitical, economic, psychological, cultural, and organizational components that affect the behaviors and the attitudes of each group. Access is a concept so broadly based as to be concerned not only with the initiation of care based on need, but also with the continuation of that care if it is needed and prescribed.[1]

Problems encountered in relation to access to health care can be defined in relation to the interaction between two systems or environments. The consumer in becoming a patient does so with his problems, desires, and needs and that human constellation "interacts with the human constellation in the health care delivery system which is composed of a variety of subsystems. . . ."[2] These include medical practitioners, nurses, administrators, social workers, and a range of other professional, paraprofessional and voluntary personnel, which have been described as representing more than 50 different occupational statuses.[3]

Before there is any interaction between an individual and a provider, the individual needs to cross a threshold. Crossing a medical threshold requires an individual to perceive a need for the available services. In looking first at the individual, the concept of "perceived need," is lodged in the attitude of the prospective user. There are many potential impediments between recognition of need and the active seeking of professional assistance, regardless of the locus of care. Once having acknowledged that the "need" may require more than self-ministration, another range of potential barriers must be overcome to cross the threshold of health services. The would-be patient faces provider attitudes and behaviors that, derive from internal forces, external influences, and structural and organizational factors. These factors, if reconciled in a mutually responsive way, should facilitate the initiation and the continuation of care, if needed. Within the last two decades, we have become more and more aware that client and provider systems may have differing perspectives of what should happen between them, what is needed and expected, and each one's responsibilities. The more complex the organization, the more complex the processes of care will be, although complications in starting care and in following medical recommendations are not limited to the complexity of the health care system.

Background

Between World War I and the early 1960's, little consideration was given to the issue of access to health and social welfare agencies. During those years, most service organizations focused attention on those who crossed the threshold. Two prevailing attitudes governed this practice. One was more or less the point of view "seek and you shall find," leaving the responsibility to know of and to act in his own behalf solely to the individual or his family. The second was the interpretation and belief held by most providers that "crossing the threshold" was an expression by the would-be client of his motivation to use the service he had sought. This was seen as the client having a "perceived need," his identification of a helping source, and seeking that help. If clients failed to use the service, once having passed the entryway or the gatekeepers of the organization, the problem in not continuing with prescribed care was seen as theirs, not that of the providers who saw themselves as available to those who sought them out. There were few, if any, efforts to "find" those—the poor, elderly, uninformed, and others—who for whatever reason were obstructed in seeking what they needed, or to hold those who had initiated care and required ongoing services but who had "dropped out."

Prior to World War I when the settlement house movement was active, the emphasis on those "in need" was different. Social welfare and health resources were limited. Yet, in spite of these limitations, individuals "at risk" (children, in particular) were the interest of reformers in the public health, mental health, or public welfare movements. These reformers—doctors, nurses, social workers and interested lay persons—moved into poor communities, sweatshop industries, and child labor factories "finding" clientele "in need" and then drawing them into the locations where existing help was available.

The 1960s brought in an era of consumer rights and student "democracy," and concern with the quality of the environment, human services, and societal benefits. Advances in medical technology and promises from physicians of more than they could actually deliver surfaced. Legislation eased financial accessibility for the elderly (Title 18, Medicare) and the poor (Title 19, Medicaid) but affected the level of demand and greatly increased the costs of health services. Failures in the provision of services to given populations by the systems of human services were seen as social deprivations of entitlement or of rights, and as chaotic "non-systems" of care. The trend by physicians toward more super-specialization and their own "good life" made access even more difficult and caused inappropriate use of available health facilities. Because the house call became a thing of the past, for such reasons as personal fear, costs, and immovable technological equipment, emergency rooms of hospitals became the medical service arena for not only the poor but also for those in real or imagined crises. Also public and voluntary health policy continued to favor hospitalized patients and as a result of the Hill-Burton Act support for the building of more hospital beds was generous. Soon these beds were either inappropriately used or empty, again adding to the acceleration of costs of care.

The incredible and affluent sixties ushered in a wave of human rights expectations and a demand for services for all of us and, in particular, the poor and deprived. Soon the results were a financial hodge-podge for medical care, a breakdown in most health care systems, and an alienation in health care providers and workers from the system and consumers. Serious gaps in the quality of care delivered and in professional accountability were apparent. Finally, there was a great outcry from the public press to correct the wrongs. Special interest groups reached politicians to attempt change.

In recent years, in addition to the outcry about the problems in the delivery of care, there is now a major concern as to whether there is equitable distribution of resources, and whether there is equity of opportunity, i.e., the same availability and the same potential accessibility irrespective of social class, economic factors, racial, religious, or educational background. Also, there are those who argue that medical services are not highly correlated with the health status of the public. This group wants to politicize public expenditures to secure better housing stock and air and water pollution controls; conquer hunger; teach good nutritional habits; and support better education for all. The arguments are that it is in the improvement of these resources that a healthy environment and a healthy public are more readily achieved than in vast expenditures for medical care.

These arguments are attacks on values and ethics in regard to serving the public good. When one addresses individuals and their perception of health maintenance, there is no question that they argue for an available and accessible medical care system but one which permits them equal access to it regardless of economic considerations. The individual represented in the "public" believes that what is currently available is not adequate nor sufficient to allow for "equity in distribution." For whatever reason John Q. Public believes that medical care can and does contribute to bettering his state of health, despite his complaints about it, and he wants it available to him.[4]

The public demand for medical care is a factor in public policy governing "how much," "what," "at what costs," "by whom," "for whom," and "where." While there is no "right to health," there is a growing conviction about the "right to health care" without limitations or rationing. While our political representatives may worry about costs, neither the consumer nor the provider does except in relation to his perception of those who are "unworthy." In any event, for all practical purposes, care is rationed by virtue of a range of barriers that affect access to it. The rationing interrelates with constraints governing income, distribution, availability, organizational, psychological, and geographic accessibility—factors that are internal to the provider system, patient system, or both, and those that may reside in the broad sociopolitical systems of society.

Barriers

Access to care requires available medical resources. Until the 1960s no regulations governed availability. In 1965, the "reasonable cost plus" reimbursement program of the government to hospitals for care of the insured permitted such an explosion in hospital facilities that by the seventies regulations were promulgated that dealt essentially with cost containment. However, no government regulation constrains the physician. Freedom to practice anywhere has been the "right" of licensed physicians so that their private practices, whether solo or group, allows them to open offices on their own terms. This means that physicians can practice the kind of medicine they wish, allocate their resources as they see fit, and set fees governed essentially on "what the traffic will bear." The impact, therefore, is that doctors may, by and large, serve whom they wish in their own offices. In this way, private medicine controls the "market to a substantial degree, administering price, quantity and quality."[5] No regulations are placed on physicians other than the required license to practice. While they may not have total control over their provision of care, they have a great deal, even to escaping the usual marketplace competition common to other entrepreneurs.

The issue of access is governed by a physician's predilections, as well as that of the medical establishment. Specialization is usually endorsed by medical educators, both by their educational direction and their traditional biases. Thus primary care services, which have been demonstrated to be the public's greatest need, are the least available. Seventy-five percent of visits made to physicians are for supportive, counseling, or caring services and are not for highly specialized needs.[6] Thus the marketplace of medicine, if services are available, may well be over-priced and offered by over-educated professionals. It is well known that most young physicians wish to continue relationships with good teaching hospitals. Thus their practices are more likely to be in urban centers containing teaching establishments rather than in rural areas or inner-city ghettos. Since most physicians as a group come from middle and upper social classes, they tend to wish to practice in relation to their own class, claiming it is easier to do so. This aspect of self-determination by physicians, a commonly held tenet in our society, has lead to a maldistribution of resources, and this affects access.

The organization of hospitals and other health care facilities can be critical in the way it affects access to services. Most of these organizations have their services organized around the needs of the people who provide the services rather than around those who receive the care. Factors that govern access to these institutions are geographic location, timing of service programs, and structural arrangements of care, along with the gatekeepers to the services.

The geographic location of a medical institution influences not only the client in his use patterns but also provider behaviors as, for example, in the way they may draw on other resources, based on proximity and distance from their own offices. While location may not affect all prospective patients equally, it is known to affect the accessibility of lower income groups. Private medical care, whether in private solo or group practices or in institutions, is generally timed during the usual business-hour obligations of prospective users. The hours in which services are offered obviously affects those who may not have free use of time. Those who cannot use daytime services must resort to institutional emergency rooms. These users compete with clients with real emergencies for evening and nighttime services of medical centers. Since the advent of Medicare and Medicaid as financial aid to the elderly and the poor, "Medicaid Mills" have emerged in urban ghettos, many of which offer a range of services in evening hours. Frequently, these types of services tend to be more sensitive to local preferences and needs than more traditional medical care systems.

Organizational arrangements can be very significant in regard to access. The doorways people enter are usually prescribed by social class. Welfare patients tend to enter through clinic and emergency room facilities while private patients enter hospitals through other doorways. This "two-class" medical care system exists in almost all medical institutions in the country. Racial segregation tends to be economically determined and nonwhites are found more frequently in the clinic system of care. Providers who treat patients in clinic areas are themselves different in race and class from those whom they serve.[7] Who monitors the doorways and how it is done can affect who remains for care. Depersonalization, common in large organizations, can be a deterrent.

The most significant barrier to access is economic. Access is highly correlated with the costs of services. Although the majority of the population is covered for some portions of medical services through different types of insurance, the degree of coverage varies considerably. It is well known that financial barriers force people to make choices not only from among the medical care resources available, but also in postponing medical care for such other needs as housing, food, and clothing. Who pays for care and how and when may be factors that encourage the use of services or act as deterrents to care. Cost, which is borne by an individual and the family versus some social instrumentality that is either governmentally or occupationally supported, may be significant. Care that is prepaid or must be concurrently paid for, either in full or as a deductible with co-payment, can be factors in affecting access. It is also known that even if financial difficulties are removed, it does not mean that the service becomes available, nor even that people will use what is available. People's behaviors, living habits, and their environment may affect what they do more than guaranteed access.[8]

Perceived Need

Who gets into the health care system is governed not only by the barriers to care already suggested, but also by whether an individual perceives a need for the specialized services of the medical care establishment. This usually involves a process that takes most individuals through many stages before they turn to the expert for help.

The dictionary offers the definition of "access" as the "right to enter or make use of." The definition implies that the individual is at the entry to the service and faces crossing the threshold. It does not consider whether the need for care has been "perceived." Perceiving the need for professional care is the *sine qua non* in seeking it.

For most individuals, beginning signs or symptoms of a disturbance in well-being are cared for through an informal system where the first step may be to ignore them, assuming they are transitory. A second may be to self-doctor, drawing on the resources of neighborhood pharmacists or family members or friends. As symptoms persist, it is then still the client who must arrive at a determination to seek professional consultation. Therefore, most often the individual must activate the consumer of services role. This is achieved when the need is recognized and actions relevant to the symptoms experienced lead the individual into a patient-of-the-doctor status.[9]

Having come to a determination to use professional services and having reached the doorway of the service, an individual faces two additional components in relation to access to care: ability to initiate entry (initiation) and ability to continue care, if prescribed (continuation).[10]

Entry and Initiation

Initiating services or attempting to cross the threshold of care-giving services can also be fraught with impediments. The organization of the care and the pathways to reach it are critical. How the medical establishment, whether private practitioner or institution, appears to a client at the doorway and in subsequent encounters can govern the quality of the interaction between consumer and provider. A critical factor is the gatekeeper at the entryway. Most private practitioners believe they serve as the first and primary encounter with their patients, forgetting that others also open the doors and steer people to professional services. This pattern is true for institutional care as well.

The single most important component of access is entry into a medical system. The ability to initiate entry is critical. An institution has a responsibility to know who crosses the threshold and be responsive to their needs, but it must also be responsible for knowing who did not get in and why. There is an indication that many of those who attempt to cross the mental health doorways are referred elsewhere or turned away. These "revolving doors" are under the jurisdiction of gatekeepers who require "passwords" for admission to their mental health centers. The "passwords" may be imposed by the doorkeepers or be a translation of providers' decisions about who is to be served. When prospective clients are referred elsewhere, there is very little in the way of followup to learn if the client has reached the next doorway. Interestingly, providers claim that when an individual has "crossed the threshold" he has demonstrated motivation for help. Yet, providers frequently place the burden on clients to find the "appropriate" or "responsive" service. Many people believe that it is an institution's responsibility to maximize a client's initiation into care and, if prescribed and appropriate, continued care within that institution or elsewhere.

The process of entry is achieved only through a reduction in or elimination of barriers to access. The entryway needs to be clearly what it is, a single doorway, undifferentiated as to individuals with different presenting problems.[11] It cannot be left to the sick to "sort" out the appropriate doorways. If there are different entryways, then clear and prompt rechanneling after entry must exist. Entries require systemized feeder systems which include screening and triage so as to uncover patients' need and locate the appropriate sources of help.[12] Careful screening permits clarification of need and is the first step in informed and clear channeling of patients to appropriate services. Those who do the screening and channeling need to be knowledgeable about resources available within the system. In order to consider a quality access system at the entry to care, Donabedian has suggested the following:

"(a) Least friction entry;
(b) Single-point, undifferentiated entry;
(c) Alternative-point entry;
(d) Formally and informally organized multiple-feeder entry;
(e) Selective and differentiated continuation of care."[13]

Once the problem and the need have been uncovered, a centralized information and referral system is required to safeguard relevant channeling to predetermined and accessible resources within the setting, if prescribed, or to an appropriate resource outside the setting. An information and referral service that translates the need and becomes the interactor between client and provider systems could be under the aegis of a patient representative program, committed to serving patients. Access implies not only an understanding of the need and knowledge of the resources but also the know-how to deal with requests.

Channeling and Continuation of Care

A basic component of access is continuation of the care initiated, regardless of location. That care, when prescribed, may take place on an outpatient or inpatient basis and may be continued into a post-hospital period, either in private or institutionally-based facilities. "The proof of access is use of service, not simply the presence of a facility."[14] Access means not only the entry into the health care system, but continuation of care.

The general hospital, as an outpatient or inpatient facility, is one of the most highly stratified and rigid of formal organizations. Hospitals have a complex labor system, ranging from super-specialists to unskilled workers, each group with its own description and functions. Medical care is traditionally based on a one-to-one intervention system. In it there is a range of professional and paraprofessional personnel: multiple specialists, technicians, aides, each of whom "lays on hands." This complicated system of division of labor results in multidepartmentalized subsystems, with autonomous department chiefs and their staffs. Each of these subsystems has its own experts, goals, and priorities. Each subsystem has its own procedures, time scheduling, and special personnel predilections and task expectations. The issue of interdependence is somewhat forced on each and neither coordination nor collaboration has high priority. If the hospital is large, complex, and part of a teaching and research center (present day mergers make this more probable than ever), then physicians may have to face the priority they will undertake—patient care, teaching or research—reflecting their own autonomous interests.

Further separations are not limited to functional responsibilities but to relationships as well. In traversing the health care system one can see the patterns of relationships: doctors relating to doctors but not to aides, the medical board to physicians and their interests, administration to the hotel services personnel and very little to physicians, the lay board ostensibly to both the medical and administrative areas, but in practice usually to neither except when there are major problems. There is little relatedness of these areas of responsibility to the comprehensiveness of care. In this atmosphere, safeguarding continuation of care as well as continuity with the same physician requires special programmatic approaches within the institution. Complex systems need an organizational flow that guarantees coordination through sound channeling.

Coordination and continuity of care need to be addressed for the short-term, immediate need, so that an individual is not caught among the fragmented parts of the large institution. Some medical centers have begun to address the long-term needs of patients and their families by establishing relationships between them and their caretakers on a stable and ongoing basis. Personalization of care, along with continuity, is what patients are seeking. Where services can be coordinated and centralized with fewer personnel rather than more, stability seems to be protected. Apart from channeling responsibilities assigned to given personnel, some medical centers have designed small units of service with stable personnel who hold responsibility for the coordination of care of each assigned patient. These units have taken the position that patients should not be expected to have to coordinate their own service requirements.

Where programs have begun to emphasize long-term care responsibility to patients, they provide periodic workups, and the assessment and ongoing needs are openly shared between patient and provider so as to safeguard continuity as well helping patients to meet medical recommendations. Continuation of care requires quality linkages within the institution. Clear records that are available on demand and good communication among responsible providers are essential. All these are necessary for professional responsibility and accountability.

Donabedian has suggested that "—access to care and insufficient use of service are legitimate elements in assessing the quality of the client-practitioner transaction as well as of the program as a whole. Insufficient access and use need special and continuing attention because so many programs are obsessively preoccupied with curbing utilization and cutting costs, even though they may pay lip service to the importance of eliminating insufficient care." He also follows the above with "excessive use of service usually means poor quality for a variety of reasons. For one it

implies a lack of skill in the conduct of patient care; an inability to proceed
from step to step along the most direct path, selecting the precisely necessary and sufficient procedures to arrive at a diagnosis and to institute
treatment."[15]

Guaranteed Access

One approach toward dealing with individuals who could fall between the internal cracks in the service organization is to develop ways
to guarantee access within the system. In order to casefind for given
services those factors that reflect "risk" or "need" will have to be determined by the potentially helping service. The casefinding or screening
approach had its beginnings in the welfare, mental health, and public
health movements when the poor, the tuberculous, the mentally ill, and
working children were of special concern to the reform-minded. Those
who were "high social risks" were identifiable by their so-called visible
characteristics.

In their search for indicators, social workers in the health system
have turned to approaches that could systematically identify "need" or
"high social risk." These attempts are predicated on the premise that all
individuals who enter a health care system with illness or disability have
social dysfunctioning associated with that disorder.[16] In addition to the
impact on social functioning and the limitations associated with illness,
the social and cultural orientation of people will affect their motivation
and capacity to follow the medical regimen. The social impact needs to
be understood and to be dealt with by the treating health care professionals
so that comprehensive care can be safeguarded. Sensitivity to social factors
in the individual can influence the outcome of services. While all those
who are "sick" may not need professional social work services, those at
high social risk do need to be found as early as possible.

Public health specialists (and some institutionally-based physicians)
have placed their emphases outside of the medical establishment in seeking
people who may have incipient or advanced problems. Their major concentration has been largely in the schools, seeking children at physical or
social risk and then referring them for needed services.

Individual Motivation

Continuation of care rests on the same set of dynamics that set the
initial process going. The key factor of motivation lies in the process of
fulfilling the contract between client and provider. Compliance with
recommendations in continuing care, such as following medical advice,
has been studied by students of motivation with the hope that understand-

ing could lead to improved response from patients who have seen physicians.[17] "While reported compliance rates do differ, they are almost uniformly low enough to indicate that a serious problem exists."[18] There is no question that by and large all patients need to act on their own behalf in following medical advice and in continuing care. The degree and the type of responsibility that individuals will take varies in accordance with a wide range of psychological and social factors. Advice that calls for changes in personal habits or in usual living styles, or that does not "fit" with the cultural pattern of the individual may well be ignored. Other situations that may interfere with patients' pursuit of care are: advice given when patients are experiencing tension or having unfavorable relationships with members of the provider system; complex instructions, regimens, and expectations; the providers ignoring patients and talking "at" them with no feedback between patients and providers; conflicting communications from providers; or unsatisfactory experiences with medical care. It is interesting that most studies reveal no definite findings which link sociodemographic factors with compliance except for the underutilization of health care facilities by the poor and minority groups. In addition, Cauffman found in her study of referrals to services and the outcomes for consumers that "if consumers showed for care, they were likely to receive care."[19] A critical interest in receiving care was a determining factor that prompted people to go for care—what motivated them. Again sociodemographic factors were not positive determinants in whether people crossed the medical threshold.

Corollary problems that had been considered significant deterrents to access were "lack of transportation, no parking, inconvenient service hours, waiting time at providers' places of service, no one to care for children, lack of financial resources and limited English competencies. Surprisingly, none of these corollary problems was significantly related to whether consumers showed for care. In fact consumers showed for care in spite of corollary problems."[20] In addition, neither time nor distance were significant factors. The variables most associated with showing for care were "consumers who were referred for health care and who received appointments with providers were much more likely to show than were consumers who did not receive appointments. Also, consumers who were referred for health care and who were given the name of a person to see were much more likely to show than were those who were not given the name of a person to see."[21] The implications of this study clearly are that there is a need for personalization of the referral at both ends—screening and receiving—to include appointments with named individuals.

Other factors will also affect the way people reach out to services, continue with care, and comply with and follow advice. These are largely provider-controlled factors: clear communication, listening to patients, securing feedback, being knowledgeable about one's patients as individuals, letting patients repeat recommendations to be sure they've been understood, simplifying the regimens so that they are compatible with patients' life styles and beliefs, and either inviting patients to return or following-up by telephone to show interest in their state of health. Again, all these bespeak to the personalization of care. The most significant factors in safeguarding access are lodged in the attitudes and behaviors of the gatekeepers and the providers, and in the motivation of the patient to act.

Gathering Information and its Feedback

To be knowledgeable about a system of care, what it provides, by whom, when and where, and at what cost requires periodic information gathering. Data about who crosses the threshold, what is presented and received, and who does not get care need to be gathered as well. This type of information can show service delivery and utilization patterns. While it does not deal with the outcome of care to patients, it does evaluate what is given and who gets what. The impediments can be identified and the problems clarified as data are analyzed and projections of alternatives made to correct the difficulties. However, "putting information to use" is not without its complications, and will be addressed more fully in the concluding chapter of this text.

It is important to consider that those individuals involved in patients' access to care be guided by more than an informal system. While the informal system, which permits information to move both up and down as well as horizontally, it also allows the attitudes and biases to move unchecked and uninformed in the same patterns. In addition, the informal system of communication will not generate change. It may even block change if there is no informed translation of need. It tends to be adaptive and not creative. A formal feedback system requires a formal communication system that is participatory in nature. Feedback to the involved and interaction with the findings can be the first steps toward an understanding of the problems and communication about them. If staff members are encouraged to participate, then a form of internal advocacy can be generated to overcome the barriers and impediments to delivery.

Whether the organization delivering the care is composed of a large number or small number of units, they "are social units consisting of a network of relations which orients and regulates the behavior among a specific set of individuals in the pursuit of relatively specific goals."[22] "Goals are only conceptions of desired ends. If they are to have consequences for the behavior of organizational participants—they must become operative; they must be translated into specific tasks which are allocated to participants. A task is simply a set of activities to achieve some goal. The end product of performing a task is an outcome."[23] The translation from goal to task to outcome may not correspond with the desired expectation. Goals, tasks and outcomes may have no interrelationship. To achieve behavioral expectations requires the investment of many people.

The intent of a feedback system is to give those involved in care a "voice" in the way the care is delivered. There are many ways to approach informed data gathering and the analyses of that data. Those responsible can carry out periodic reviews of given areas on a rotated basis. Some people suggest that the review can take place when problems are already reported. The former approach may preclude the latter; however, whenever a major problem surfaces, the area should be reviewed. Periodic reviews allow for assessment of a program's effectiveness. By drawing on those involved, reviews permit a sharing as well as a dissemination of information and knowledge. It is a way of having staff members contribute to their own wish to change. It is well-demonstrated that superimposed decision-making, without a staff's investment generally eliminates both the rationale or incentive to do anything differently.

Securing a staff's advocacy for change helps to sustain commitment to the basic purposes of the program. Administrative support for staff involvement in practice, not in words only, tends to motivate the staff's interest. Keeping the staff informed and involved through a feedback on the review of given programs allows those involved to see what happens as a result of their activities. It develops an awareness of the problem, a sense of felt need, a recognition that something needs to be done about it, and a willingness to get involved. When done in a nonpunitive way to stimulate recognition and initiative, a staff tends to become invested in the need.

All organizations need a self-examining system that has problem-uncovering and problem-solving mechanisms. However they are designed, they are intended to detect a problem, analyze it, develop resolution ideas, then open discussion and choice among those who will be most affected by any change. The change program needs to be developed. It can be implemented only when good orientation and training are introduced. Then periodic assessment of how the new system is working is essential in order to give the staff involved a chance to "de-bug" and make improvements. There are no ways to hurry-up the process of participation in improving service delivery.

Conclusions

Access is the most critical dynamic operative in the health care system. An individual has to get in before he gets care and then he needs to continue within that system, if recommended, or reach another system of services. The effectiveness of access is lodged in two major systems: the individual and the provider, with all the complexities of social, environmental, economic, cultural, psychological, and organizational influences. Access means crossing a threshold. Before one reaches the doorway, he needs to recognize a need and to act on it by seeking professional assistance. Acting means that the individual is able to overcome the barriers to care. In reaching the doorway, initiation of care must occur. Unless care is initiated there can be no continuation. Access requires motivation to respond by the prospective user, and motivation to serve by the prospective provider, whether it is for directly administered services or is indirect by informing and referring the individual in need to an appropriate facility. Access is rationed by virtue of the constraints arising out of economic, distributive, organizational, and individual human behavioral factors. Barriers are imposed by providers and their organizations, as well as by the limitations in public policy. Does access mean equitable distribution of medical care services and equity of opportunity to use them by all sectors of the population? At this time there are arguments for social policy that permit the same availability and accessibility irrespective of socioeconomic facts. The public is asking for this, and there are indications that they are willing to pay for equity. The difficulty is in finding the definition for the "right to health care."

A major problem in achieving successful access is a growing depersonalization and fragmentation of care. A new personal commitment to serving those who are ill is what is sought. What does commitment to giving care require? How is personalized and sound care achieved? While no single professional can carry solo responsibility for the process from beginning through on-going in the short run or over the long term, an overall consciousness of the objectives of the program of care is essential in each person who works with patients, along with a commitment to the specific tasks assigned.

It is not enough to know only the tasks. They need to be understood in the context of program objectives for patients. How one enters the system, the flow of service, their initiation and continuation, channeling and coordination, along with the quality of terminating care are critical knowledge factors for all personnel who "lay on hands." For those who are close to individual patients offering clinical services, in addition to an awareness of self as a practicing health care professional or paraprofessional, an understanding of the people who use or will use the services both as individuals and as a member of a given population group is essential. This means some understanding of behavioral dynamics. Programs need to be developed that are perceived "in behalf of patients' needs." This calls for a conscious awareness of the structure, its personnel environment and its organizational environment, and how it can and does affect the providers in the way they give care.

It is important to recognize that "better" health care and delivery will generate the uncovering of more illness. If people are seen and diagnosed, their problems are perceived and they have not postponed entry into a medical care system. Donabedian suggests that an effective system has a "discovery effect" because it "reveals and records previously undiagnosed or reported illnesses."[24] Therefore, a factor in access includes an effective system of outreach and good entry, so as to safeguard screening and casefinding of those with need. Access is also dependent on the public as well as on the individual in what he does or does not do for himself. There is no question that without motivation and self-investment no health gains can be realized by the individual. On the other hand, the elderly, the poor, minorities, and others cannot be blamed for not responding to opportunities not open to them. Access is affected by the distribution and the accessibility of health care services. However, where the problems are in different population groups is a critical factor in whether services should be designed to meet those needs and to encourage access to them. At the current time most health care services are designed with a concentration on the disease or the organ affected, for example, multiple sclerosis specialist or orthopedic service.

To make the delivery of care effective, the provider system and the individual (and his family) need to be linked to each other in some other way than at present. In addition to achieving availability of resources and the willingness and interest to deal with individuals and what they need, a system of care needs to be committed to a "democracy" of services to people. This means an open system, willing to review what and how it practices, who it serves and who it does not; willing to involve the staff in assessment and in advocacy for change, and open to the introduction of innovative interventions, even risk-taking in how it safeguards sound care to those who need it.

References

1. Avedis Donabedian. "Models for Organizing the Delivery of Personal Health Services and Criteria for Evaluating Them." In *Organizational Issues in the Delivery of Health Services.* Edited by I.K. Zola and J.B. McKinley, Prodist, New York, 1974, p. 135.

2. Richard Beckhard. "Organizational Issues in the Team Delivery of Comprehensive Health Care." In Zola and McKinley, *Op. cit.,* p. 99.

3. Herbert E. Klarman. *The Economics of Health,* Columbia University Press, New York, 1965, p. 4.

4. Rashi Fein. "On Achieving Access and Equity in Health Care" in *Medical Cure and Medical Care.* Edited by Spyros Andreapoulos, *The Milbank Memorial Fund Quarterly* 50: 4: 157–190, Oct. 1972, Part 2, Prodist, New York.

5. *Ibid.,* p. 176.

6. Lewis Thomas. "On the Science and Technology of Medicine." *Daedalus* Winter 1977, p. 42.

7. Donabedian. *Op. cit.,* pp. 154–156.

8. *Ibid.* pp. 156–158.

9. Avedis Donabedian. *Aspects of Medical Care Administration.* Harvard University Press, Cambridge, Mass., 1973, pp. 58–59.

10. Donabedian. *Op. cit.* In Zola and McKinley, p. 135.

11. *Ibid.* p. 135.

12. *Ibid.* p. 136.

13. *Ibid.* p. 136.

14. *Ibid.* p. 135.

15. Avedis Donabedian. "A Frame of Reference." In *Needed Research in the Assessment and Monitoring of the Quality of Medical Care.* Hyattsville, Md., National Center for Health Services Research, U.S. Department of Health, Education and Welfare, Publication No. (PHS) 78-3219, 1978, p. 2.

16. H. Rehr, B. Berkman, and G. Rosenberg. "A Social Work Department Develops and Tests a Screening Mechanism to Identify High Social Risk Situations," *Social Work in Health Care* 5:4, Summer 1980, pp. 373–385.

17. For studies reported on the subject of compliance see Milton S. Davis. *Journal of Medical Education* 41:11:1037–1048, Nov. 1966; *American Journal of Public Health* 58:2:274–288, Feb. 1968; *Medical Care* 6:2:115–122, March-April 1968; also Julia D. Watkins et al. *American Journal of Public Health* 57:3:452–459, March 1967; also Leon Gordis, et al. *Medical Care* 7:2:49–54, January-February 1969.

18. Rona Levy. "Facilitating Patient Compliance with Medical Programs" in *Social Work in Health Care.* Edited by Neil F. Bracht, The Haworth Press, New York 1978, p. 282.

19. Joy G. Cauffman, et al. "A Study of Health Referral Patterns; IV Factors Related to Referral Outcomes," *American Journal of Public Health* 64:4:353, April 1974.

20. *Ibid.* pp. 353–354.

21. *Ibid.* p. 354.

22. W. Richard Scott. "Some Implications of Organizational Theory for Research on Health Services." In Zola and McKinley, *Op. cit.,* p. 4.

23. *Ibid.* p. 8.

24. Donabedian. In Zola and McKinley, *Op. cit.,* p. 131.

Chapter II

The Current Climate in Hospital Care

MILDRED D. MAILICK

Public concern about quality of health care and access to it in and outside of hospitals has become a highly emotional national issue. This is reflected not only in the amount of space and time devoted by the media to how health care is provided but also in an escalating debate about ways in which legislation for new health care programs can be formulated so as to ensure equity of access as well as quality of care for patients at reasonable cost. It is also reflected in the growing number of regulations and programs that attempt to monitor medical care in the interests of patients.

Background

Although the predominant mode of providing medical care is still solo practice by physicians, the trend is toward physician partnerships and group practice. There has been a shift of diagnostic and treatment services in the past two decades from physicians' offices toward general hospitals. The expensive, elaborate equipment, skilled technicians, and labor intensive services of modern medical care are difficult to support in the office of an individual physician. Economies of large scale require such equipment and services be located where frequent use can justify the heavy capital investment and ongoing labor costs. Partly because they can economically support the services, general hospitals have become the locus for diagnostic testing and treatment involving a high level of technology. Thus, a hospital is no longer a place where people go only for surgery or to receive treatment for severe illness; it has expanded to include diagnostic and treatment functions that were once carried out in physicians' offices or patients' homes. Further, hospital emergency rooms have become the primary care service for the poor.

Hospitals, their medical facilities and services have become a key factor in the provision of medical care. An examination of the current hospital system and how patients enter it and receive care within it is essential in understanding the quality and equity of services.

Growth in Size and Complexity of Hospitals

Not only have general hospitals become more important in the delivery of medical care, they have become larger. Small hospitals under pressure to maintain underutilized specialties and equipment for prestige, training, or other reasons have begun to pool resources and allocate and share specialties with other hospitals in regional plans. Many of these hospitals have either merged or affiliated with larger medical centers. Between 1964 and 1974 there was a 50 percent increase in the number of general hospitals with 300 or more beds in the United States.[1] There is evidence however that the trend toward increasing size has reached its peak for the time being.[2]

Many proprietary and voluntary hospitals are in financial jeopardy because of low utilization rates. National and local officials have withdrawn their support for legislation that provides incentives for building new hospitals or for expanding the size of existing institutions. Local health planning boards have become increasingly stringent about giving approval to any increase in the number of hospital beds, especially in regions where existing hospitals are underutilized and beds stand empty. Yet any major attempt to reduce the size of hospitals by mandated closure of beds has been met by concerted resistance from the hospitals, unions and local communities. Thus, it is likely that hospital beds will remain at a stable level in the forseeable future.

In addition to changes in size, hospitals have become more complex. This is reflected by a rise in the number and kinds of specialized services offered by hospitals. Between 1961 and 1971, for example, hospitals with intensive care units increased by 63 percent. Similarly, cardiac intensive care units, which did not exist in 1961, are now found in over 2,000 hospitals.[3] The American Hospital Association lists 54 different special facilities and services in general hospitals and the larger, more complex hospitals have all of them.[4]

Each of these special facilities and services must be housed in its own specific area in the hospital and must employ technicians and specialists who have the necessary expertise to operate them. Every specialty generates its own goals and priorities, communication patterns, and optimum arrangements of work. This has led to a large number of compartmentalized hospital departments that have often been described as small fiefdoms. Though each is, to a limited extent, separate and autonomous, a degree of interdependence is forced upon them partly by their need to share the "product," that is, the patient.

The trend in hospitals toward increased size, specialization, complexity, and compartmentalization requires patients to cope with a large number of service components that tend to fragment care. While patients eagerly seek the technology and expertise of the modern hospital, it often appears to them to be a confusing maze which must successfully be negotiated in order to reach any, and sometimes life-saving, services.

Another aspect of hospital complexity is the great variety of employees in different occupational groups. No service in a modern medical center functions in the absence of other essential supplementary services. Even routine medical care requires multilevel and multidepartmental involvement. More than 50 separate occupations work together in a hospital, each with its own job description and prescribed duties. Many of these groups of people carry out their duties without direct contact with patients, but, even so, patients must deal with a surprising number of health workers and they are sometimes confused by a lack of knowledge about what each can or will do.

Health workers are governed by a set of hospital rules, and sometimes by union rules as well, which may prevent, or can be used as rationale to prevent, workers from going beyond the scope of their responsibilities when a simple request is made by patients. Very basic human needs are sometimes unattended because they seem to be no one's task. Patients' care is thus fragmented not only by the compartmentalization of the hospital function and structure but also by the tasks of the workers.

Growth in Importance of the Hospital Administrator

In addition to factors of size, complexity, and specialization, modern hospitals have slowly been changing in terms of the division of policy-making power between medical and administrative personnel. The physicians and medical boards of hospitals still wield considerable power, and little real change can occur without their agreement and cooperation. However, a shift has taken place, and physicians no longer have the unchallenged authority in hospitals they once did. Government policy, regulations of commercial and nonprofit insurance companies, a growing need for careful financial management, the power of unions, and the public's concern are among the many forces that have reduced the absolute status of physicians.[5] As a result of becoming a mediator between all of these interest groups hospital administrators have assumed a position of increased power. In addition to the interest groups within hospitals, courts have begun to hold hospitals, as corporate entities, responsible in some malpractice suits for the actions of their physicians and this has allowed hospital administrators to assert more control over doctors.[6, 7]

The implications for patients of this shift in power are not yet very clear. On the one hand, physicians acted as advocates and sometimes used leverage to get special services for their private patients. They also acted as coordinators of service and could exercise authority to cut through red tape. On the other hand, physicians often used their power in hospitals to influence the organization of services so that they became the most economic, convenient, and advantageous to them. Patients have been expected to accommodate themselves to the resulting routines of service, sometimes at the cost of considerable distress.

The relationship between administrators and patients is quite different. Administrators tend to think not in terms of individual patients, but in terms of categories of patients for whom services can be provided, evaluated, and even predicted. This view of patients as a group tends to lead to less individualization and more formalization of services. Administrators' perception of the task as including the management of both medical and nonmedical services and attending to the comfort and satisfaction of patients as consumers, however, tends to encourage the development of mechanisms to serve patients' interest.[8]

To a small extent the shift of power to administrators may increase the power of patients. If the only source of redress of grievance or change is a physician on whom a patient is dependent, then patients are less likely to complain. Research documents that patients, at least while in the hospital, are reluctant to express complaints directly to doctors and nurses.[9] If patients have avenues of complaints to those who have less obvious power to directly retaliate against them, they might be able to assert their needs more effectively.

Changes Due to Methods of Financing Medical Care

Third-party payment (government and private) to hospitals has had a significant effect on the growth of hospitals. In 1950, only 30 percent of hospital costs were paid for by third-party payments. By 1975, the figure had risen to nearly 90 percent: 35.4 percent by private health insurance carriers and 52.9 percent by government.[10] Since until recently insurance completely covered most procedures performed in hospitals but not if done on an outpatient basis, there was pressure by patients for admission to hospitals. This distorted the pattern of health care, drawing more of the health insurance income to hospitals, resulting in their overutilization and pressure on them to grow larger. Recognition of these problems has led to pilot attempts to change patterns of reimbursement, and to allow for insurance coverage of more outpatient tests, but, thus far, there has not been much change in hospital utilization.

Both government and commercial insurance have traditionally computed payment on the basis of reasonable cost of service. All hospital expenses that can be construed as directly or indirectly related to the cost of patient care have been included. The effect of this manner of reimbursement has been to allow hospitals to expand activities and services with the expectation that the major part of the costs would be picked up by third-party payers.[11] Other aspects of expansion of hospitals were financed by federal grants provided by the Hill-Burton Act. In other words, hospitals could expand, increase facilities and specialties, hire more employees, and expect a large part of the cost to be written off in patients' bills or by government funding. The average hospital expense per adjusted patient day (which is arrived at by including inpatient and outpatient costs) rose from $44 in 1964 to $260 in 1979, and continues to rise.[12]

The effect of the growth of third-party payments in hospitals has been two-fold. First, as the size and complexity of hospitals increased there has been a need for mechanisms to provide a link between the enlarged bureaucracy and individual patients. A second effect has been a rapid inflation of hospital costs. Government and nongovernmental third-party payers have begun to pressure for the monitoring of hospital expenses in the early seventies. Cost containment rather than further expansion and program innovation has become the primary concern. Along with efforts to reduce unnecessary or overly lengthy hospital stays has been a move toward monitoring the quality of care received by patients.

Societal Recognition of Patients' Rights

Just as significant changes have occurred within hospitals, important social changes in the past few decades are also important. One of these has been the considerable attention, at least on an ideological level, given to securing and extending the rights of individuals. This was expressed first by the civil rights movement of the 1960s and then later by movements for the rights of women, welfare groups, and mental patients. The "right to health" is no doubt a nebulous concept and has many practical, ethical, and philosophical ambiguities, but it has become the political and ideological foundation for the development of pressure for legislation to provide access to health care on an equitable basis and the development of a consumer movement in health.[13]

Early health consumerism began in the 1930s. It took the form of small health cooperatives, which employed physicians and other medical services, and thus exercised some control over them. Labor unions have also bargained for and gained some control over health benefits, especially by procuring for the worker the right to choose between several health plans and by conducting health education for union members.[14]

The increasing use of the term "health consumer" instead of "client" or "patient" indicates a change in perspective. These latter terms imply dependency and involve relinquishment of some autonomy to the professional. The word "consumer," on the other hand, implies a purchase of service and with it a more independent set of social relationships.[15] What is lacking is any major coalition of unions, consumer groups, and others. Nor has there been any unified expression by them about how to improve health care, how to set priorities about health care services, and how to involve consumers in some measure of control over the entire health care system.[16]

Even though health consumerism is not strong or unified, it still represents a potential threat to hospital systems. Hospitals in neighborhoods with poverty level populations, for example, sometimes developed patient representative programs in clinics or emergency rooms not only to provide better service for neighborhood residents, but also to reduce the potential for organized community demands and threats.

On a national level, the American Hospital Association has also responded to the potential impact of consumerism. In 1973, it published a model *Patient's Bill of Rights* which it recommended, but did not mandate, that its member hospitals adopt. Except in states that are required by the hospital code to adopt the *Patient's Bill of Rights,* each hospital, through its board of directors, can exercise its own judgment about accepting the model bill, rejecting it, or changing and adapting it. In general, the *Patient's Bill of Rights* contains a mixture of provisions. A number of them merely reiterate legal rights that had already been secured by federal administrative regulations and some state legislation. These include confidentiality of medical records, the right of the patient of access to his records, the right to informed consent both for medical procedures and for participation in medical experimentation, and the right to refuse treatment. Some of the provisions of the bill of rights, however, set forth vague goals for the quality of care and for the respectful treatment of patients that are difficult to define in operational terms and, therefore, difficult to enforce.

Some hospital legal departments have been unsure about the extent of liability that a hospital incurs by the adoption of the *Patient's Bill of Rights* and have recommended against it. In hospitals that have decided to commit their institutions to the *Patient's Bill of Rights,* its adoption usually requires that someone be listed as responsible for receiving complaints or inquiries that emanate from its distribution or posting. Often the patient representative is given this specific responsibility.

Changed Patient Population

There has been a considerable change in the demographic and health status of the patient population, and this has had an impact on health care services. The proportion of the elderly in the population has been steadily increasing since 1900, and now about 10 percent of the population is 65 years or older. As a group, they are better educated and more politically active than they were 75 years ago, and they also suffer from different health problems.[17] More people have survived the infectious and communicable diseases of childhood than ever before, but now are subject to the long-term chronic and catastrophic illnesses of middle and old age. About half of the population of the United States now suffers one or more chronic illness and this has changed the nature of the health services provided by hospitals.[18]

Most general hospitals, especially those in large medical centers, are set up as short-term facilities. They are not geared financially or in work routines to care for long-term patients who may need a series of hospitalizations, each with a longer stay than is required by the acute patient. The average length of stay of persons 65 years and over in short-term general hospitals is more than double that of younger patients.

While treatment of acute illness is directed toward cure, and therefore tends to be episodic, the treatment of chronic illness focuses to a larger extent on ongoing correction and palliation. In these latter cases, continuity of care is very important as many of the problems require patients to make continuing adjustments in life style and medical regimens and, further, there is need for many ancillary, nonmedical services. This kind of care is available in part from private physicians. However, a large number of the elderly, the poor, or the near poor seek care for chronic illness in hospital outpatient clinics, and periodically they become inpatients. A major problem is that they are served to a large extent by interns and residents who rotate on a monthly or quarterly basis. Thus, those most needing the continuity of services and the development of a relationship of trust are often served by a different physician at each visit.

The enactment of Titles XVIII and XIX of the Social Security Act in 1965 created the Medicare and Medicaid programs for reimbursement to hospitals and extended care facilities, not only for care of the elderly but also for the medically needy. This legislation has had a significant effect on many aspects of medical care, including the change in the relationship between the elderly and medically indigent patients and the hospital clinic or inpatient facility. While many of these patients were previously treated free of charge or at reduced rates, they now, through government reimbursement, are paying the full cost of their care. Power relations have shifted, especially in teaching hospitals; "charity" patients have become consumers with some power to choose among doctors and medical facilities. The source of training for interns and residents is thus less stable.

Power relations have shifted in an additional way. As users of health services become better educated, they become more discriminating and judgmental about their care. As a group, they are less malleable and demand more explanation and accountability. The teaching and research functions of hospitals are affected by this shift of power; the population of the poor and near poor now must be dealt with quite differently than before in order to continue to gain their cooperation.

Changes are evident in many hospitals and emphasize the shift toward greater accountability to patients. The fact that medical personnel are required to wear name tags and identify their status in some hospitals is symbolic of this change. Another reflection of the same kind is the increasing rigorousness with which hospital committees examine the protocols of research projects for fairness and safety for patients before they give approval.

Hospitals located in central cities have been especially affected by these changes. One hundred twenty of the largest academic medical centers, which have a combined budget of $12.5 billion per year, provide 30 percent of the visits of the American public to hospitals for care in emergency rooms and outpatient clinics. One quarter of these hospitals are located in decaying inner city areas and over one-half are in the 40 largest cities in the United States.[19] These hospitals have become the object of pressure from civil rights and other groups to improve medical and non-medical services to the poor.

Hospitals have often been characterized as middle-class institutions staffed with middle-class professionals and requiring such middle-class attributes of its patients as future orientation, capacity to maintain role distance during health encounters, and the ability to fill out interminable forms. The poor are often at a disadvantage in using services in these settings; sometimes they do not possess the requisite skills to effectively obtain services. Remedies lie in the direction of either changing the attitudes and skills of individuals and groups using the hospital, or changing the pattern of service in hospitals to meet the cultural and life style needs of the clientele. Both of these alternatives have met with limited success. The former approach has demonstrated repeatedly the difficulty of changing the attitudes or practices of any group in relation to health and medical care, while the latter approach has met with few permanent changes in bureaucratic structure or orientation.[20]

In addition to the aged, the chronically ill, and the poor, other special patient groups have had an impact on hospital functioning and have required special mechanisms for care. The increased utilization by minority group members of hospital services has necessitated dealing with barriers of culture and language. Children who appear to have been abused or neglected are another group who need special services along with their parents. Very often, some groups of patients fall into several categories at once. Patients may be old, poor, and also be unable to speak English and may need special help in the light of this.

Changed Expectations of Medical Care

Paradoxically, while the medical problems of the population are becoming more chronic in nature, the public still has rising expectations of the potentials for cure. Television and other media have an important influence. As knowledge of the spectacular aspects of medical discoveries and technology are disseminated in both fiction and feature stories, the public has come to expect that something can be done about any medical condition. The metaphor of the human being as a machine is commonly held. Previously, the body was perceived as a machine that could be expected to work well for a period of time but would eventually wear out. Now, more people are looking for replaceable parts and a complete over-haul from medicine and are discontented when they don't get it.

In addition, physicians are being held accountable not only for a reasonable amount of carefulness, expertise, and skill in the process of the medical encounter, but also for its outcome. As suggested by Renee Fox,

> To some extent . . . the rise in the number of malpractice suits in the United States seems not only to be a reaction to the errors and abuses that physicians can commit, but also a reflection of the degree to which the profession is being held personally responsible for the scientific and techni-cal uncertainties of their discipline. The vision of an iatrogenic-free fur-thering of health . . . is also an indicator of such rising expectations.[21]

Hospitals, similarly, are being held increasingly responsible for their activities. Patient dissatisfaction is believed to arise from the accumulation of petty grievances encountered during hospitalization and may be an underlying factor in the development of malpractice suits. The elimination of these grievances or attention to them is of growing concern to hospitals.

The relationship of hospitals to their patients has many facets and is a source of continuing complexity. To an increasing extent hospitals have become aware of the need not only to improve the technical performance of medical care, but also to attend to the milieu in which it takes place. The changing elements in the health care system point to an increased role for patients in articulating their own needs and monitoring the quality of care they receive.

The Patient as Consumer

Patients, in their own self-interest, have a potential for providing special contributions to the control of the quality and access to medical care. While they lack expertise in some areas, they are superbly qualified to assess a series of elements in health care that have received little notice by the medical profession. It is the patients' own convenience, physical and emotional comfort, and sometimes their very survival to which they, above all, are acutely attuned. While they may not possess the expert knowledge to make medical judgments and often lack emotional objectivity, they can be, and are, a most interested and involved constituency in evaluating health care.

Self interest by patients is not a new posture; nor is the difficulty they have had in expressing concerns about their care. Even when most medical encounters took place between one physician and one patient, when more nursing care was provided at home, and when many patients paid for their medical care by direct payment, there were relatively few ways in which patients could express their preferences and dissatisfactions. Under some circumstances there was the ultimate freedom to choose among physicians and hospitals. In the main, however, patients have been strikingly powerless consumers who have had little voice in their own care. The freedom to choose among physicians has often been illusory, limited by the paucity of physicians in many communities, by lay persons' lack of confidence in their capacity to judge medical care, by the socialization in our society of both health care providers and patients to reciprocal authoritarian and subservient roles, and, in the case of the poor, by having to accept what was provided for them as charity.

It is only in the past 10 or 15 years that patients' interest has been voiced at all by individual patients. Local and federal legislators have been ambivalent and inconsistent in promoting patients' interests. Domination by the medical profession has been overwhelming. It has tended to define public policy and retard legislative action at all levels of government in relation to monitoring the quality of care. Some progress is exemplified by the Partnership for Health Act (1966), which set the climate for health providers and consumers to deliberate together about local health problems, and, more recently (1974), the establishment of the Health Systems Agencies which, while still provider dominated, allows lay consumers some voice in health policy.

In spite of these nominal increases in the influence of consumers in shaping public policy, considerable difficulty remains in their ability to affect medical encounters at the personal level. Patients feel isolated and vulnerable, and are intimidated and afraid to assert themselves. Especially in hospitals, patients are under stress and feel dependent on the staff. In many respects, the position of patients has worsened in the last few decades. Medical encounters have become less personal. Patients must contend with many more technicians and other personnel in their quest for health service. Patients do not have direct choice in the selection of technicians, who in turn, do not consider themselves directly accountable to patients. Hospital patients may hesitate to express their reactions to what they perceive as errors or failure to provide services. Patients are unsure about what the consequences may be and are fearful of retaliation. Communication is thus impeded, and patients may allow their dissatisfaction with the care to assume major proportions before they complain. Then the complaint that is made may be about an incident that has only symbolic significance and represents only a part of the real dissatisfaction. Obstacles to communication also contribute to misperceptions and misunderstandings by patients about hospital procedures that on the surface appear insensitive to their needs or feelings, but which hospitals may consider medically necessary or else required to organize work effectively. Some mechanism seems indicated by which patients' disproportionate lack of power and difficulty in communicating is ameliorated without reducing their chances of getting good medical care.

To some extent, the increase in medical malpractice suits against physicians and hospitals is a reflection of the problem of an individual's power relationship with medical personnel and hospitals. However, redress of grievance by legal means requires that damage must occur before a remedy is applied; this is, to say the least, an ineffective way for patients to affect the quality of the care. It is also an ineffective way for health care providers to respond to patient complaints.

Summary

We are currently struggling with problems that result from changes in the health care system. An upheaval has taken place in the relationship between providers and consumers. The binding ties between physicians and patients have been weakened, and in some socioeconomic groups have been virtually destroyed. Even under circumstances where solo private practitioners are available to segments of society, there is growing recognition that their capacity to provide comprehensive medical care has been reduced by fragmentation, the patterns of financial reimbursement, specialization, and complexity of the available health services. The use of a private physician as provider, coordinator, and evaluator of service to an individual patient is not only costly and time consuming, but is also increasingly less successful. The alienated consumer of health and medical services therefore faces mounting problems in gaining access to appropriate care and assessing its quality.

The estrangement of patients from providers of health and medical care was initially conceptualized as a problem of consumers. Studies of utilization patterns explored the influence of psychological, social, cultural, and economic factors on the decision-making process of individuals seeking use of medical service. "Health behavior" was the focus of attention, and remedies posed were basically intended to change the motivation or the actions of patients. Recognition of the "external" factors of availability, acceptability, and financial accessibility of health services led to a more complex formulation of the problem. Health care utilization is now recognized as a multidimensional and, as yet, poorly understood phenomenon. The search for new mechanisms for alleviating the problems of access, utilization, and evaluation of health and medical care leads to a dual focus on the system and individuals.

A body of literature has developed that suggests that when individuals have difficulty in intervening on their own behalf in large bureaucracies, such as hospitals, it does not necessarily denote an incapacity or defect within the person. Hospital bureaucracies are seen as large and powerful, governed by implacable and, at times, frustrating rules, and possessing resources and expertise far beyond those of the individual. The inequality of status is heightened in a hospital bureaucracy because patients lack expert knowledge about the services being sought and cannot rely upon market mechanisms to monitor choice. In addition, they seek entry to hospitals at a point of crisis when concern about health problems increases their vulnerability.

The mechanisms described in the next five chapters have as their purpose the linking of individuals with the complex health bureaucracy. Information and referral services provide information, advice, channeling, referral, advocacy, and/or follow-up services that help prospective patients identify and locate appropriate health services as well as to determine eligibility for their use.

Community-based health ombudsmen and advocacy programs are usually freestanding programs sponsored by consumers and community or professional groups. They serve as another link between an individual and the hospital. While often providing information and referral, their major function is to respond to complaints and grievances made by patients about the availability, acceptability, and the quality of care provided by the health bureaucracy. Both of these mechanisms help prospective patients reach the threshold of the hospital. Once inside, patients may need continued help in obtaining appropriate service. Patient representative programs fulfill part of this need. These programs attempt to identify and resolve obstacles in the hospital that affect the quality and acceptability of patient care.

All of these mechanisms have one common characteristic: they start with the patient. In contrast to social policy or bureaucratic measures, which legislate programs at a macro level, these programs deal with people who somehow are not getting the services intended for them. They start with the expressed needs, wishes, or problems of those who need medical care. They speak for patients and act as their advocates.

References

1. American Hospital Association. *Hospital Statistics.* 1975 Edition, (Chicago: American Hospital Association. 1975), p. ix.

2. United States Department of Health, Education and Welfare. *The Nation's Use of Health Resources. 1979* DHEW Publication (PHS) 80-1240, p. 52.

3. John Knowles. "The Hospital," *Life and Death and Medicine, A Scientific American Book.* San Francisco: W.H. Freeman and Company, 1973, p. 96.

4. American Hospital Association. *Hospital Statistics.* 1975 Edition, *Op. cit,* p. 187.

5. Eli Ginsberg. "Health Services, Power Centers and Decision-Making Mechanisms." *Daedalus* 106:1:204, Winter 1977.

6. F. Darling v. Charlestown Community Memorial Hospital. 33III. 2nd, 326, 211 N.E. 2d 253 (1965), cert. denied, 383 U.S. 946 (1966).

7. George F. Annas. *The Rights of Hospital Patients.* An American Civil Liberties Union Handbook. New York: Avon Books, 1975, p. 21.

8. Richard Scott. "Professionals in Hospitals: Technology and the Organization of Work." *Organization Research on Health Institutions.* Edited by Basil S. Georgopoulos, Ann Arbor: Institute for Social Research, University of Michigan, 1972, pp. 151–155.

9. Daisy M. Tagiacozzo and Hans A. Mauksch. "The Patient's View of the Patient's Role." *Patients, Physicians and Illness.* Edited by E. Gartly Jaco, 2nd Edition New York: Free Press, 1972, pp. 172–175.

10. Report to Congress. *Health, United States, 1975,* United States Department of Health, Education and Welfare (H.E.W. Publication No. HRA 76-1232), p. 27.

11. Dorothy P. Rice. "Financing Social Welfare: Health Care." *Encyclopedia of Social Work,* Sixteenth Issue, Vol. I. Edited by Robert Morris, et al. New York: National Association of Social Workers, 1971, p. 437.

12. Craig Coclen and Daniel Sullivan. "An Analysis of the Effects of Prospective Reimbursement Programs on Hospital Expenditures." *Health Care Financing Review* 2:3:1, Winter 1981.

13. Daniel Callahan. "Health and Society: Some Ethical Imperatives." *Daedalus* 106:1:25–30, Winter 1977.

14. Lester Breslow. "Consumer-Defined Goals for the Health Care Systems of the 1980s." *Technology and Health Care Systems of the 1980s.* Proceedings of a Conference, January 19–21, 1971, San Francisco, California. Edited by Morris Collen, Washington: United States Department of Health, Education and Welfare, Health Services and Mental Health Administration, 1972, p. 115.

15. Leo G. Reeder. "The Patient-Client as a Consumer: Some Observations on the

Patient-Client Relationship." *Journal of Health and Social Behavior* 13:-4:409–10, Dec. 1972.

16. Breslow. *Ibid.* pp. 116–122.

17. Bernice L. Neugarten. "Age Groups in American Society and the Rise of the Young Old." *Annals of Political and Social Sciences,* Vol. 396 (September, 1974), pp. 187–198.

18. Elihu M. Gerson and Anselm L. Straus. "Time for Living: Problems in Chronic Illness Care." *Social Policy* 6:12, Nov./Dec. 1975.

19. David E. Rogers and Robert J. Blendon. "The Academic Medical Center: A Stressed American Institution." *New England Journal of Medicine* 298:-17:940–950, April 27, 1978.

20. John B. McKinley and Diana Dutton. "Social-Psychological Factors Affecting Health Service Utilization." *Consumer Incentives for Health Care.* Edited by Selma Mushkin. New York: Prodist, 1974, pp. 251–303.

21. Renee C. Fox. "Medicalization and Demedicalization." *Daedalus* 106:1:10–11, Winter 1977.

Part II

Crossing the Hospital Threshold

Chapter III

Reaching For Care: Information and Referral Services

RISHA LEVINSON

The gaps, impediments, and inadequacies within health and social services have been well documented in the literature, with reports on problems of bureaucratic complexities, financial barriers, and restrictive admissions criteria. Inconvenient hours of service and transportation problems have further restricted access to services. Furthermore, racial and ethnic biases have compounded communication gaps, thus making entry to services more difficult for some clients. Another limitation is the tendency of the American consumer to be reluctant, and even resistive, about asking for information or requesting services lest the inquiry carry the stigma of "asking for welfare."

Specialization and fragmentation of health care services have failed to meet the multifaceted needs of the young, the old, and the chronically ill. Maldistribution of medical facilities and health personnel often make it difficult to reach services within convenient distances. Continuity of care is frequently interrupted, not only by lack of available resources but also from lack of knowledge of existing health benefits and/or health care services. The need for optimum utilization of available and appropriate resources recently has been highlighted by the increased numbers of deinstitutionalized patients returned to the community.

Titmuss has characterized the health consumer as "uniquely disadvantaged" by an inability to shop around for health services in a competitive marketplace, particularly when dealing with "life and death" situations.[1] Adequate health care, thus, is often unavailable and inaccessible, both for episodic as well as general health care.

One organizational response to overcome the many and complex barriers to medical and health care services, and to facilitate entry to needed services, is the development of information and referral services, generally referred to as "I & R."

Emergence of I and R Services

While the evolution of systematized I & R services can be traced to the central registries of clients maintained by the Social Services Exchange of one hundred years ago, it was not until the early 1960s that identifiable I & R services emerged in the public and voluntary sectors, as a result of demands for the right to access generated by consumers.

By the mid-1960s, federal legislation mandated I & R experimental programs in public health departments and in community programs for "older Americans." In response to demands for services, benefits, and entitlements by local antipoverty leaders and other advocates of the consumer rights movements, a wide variety of health and social agencies developed general and specialized I & R programs in public health clinics, community mental health centers, and community councils, as well as in store fronts and other local sites of community action programs.

Concurrently, national voluntary organizations, including the United Way, Easter Seals Society for Crippled Children and Adults, and the American Red Cross, developed information and referral programs for implementation by local chapters and affiliate membership. A variety of local volunteer groups, such as church and special interest groups, also organized I & R services for selected age groups and around such specific problems as alcoholism and drug abuse. Hotlines sprang up overnight to provide peer counseling, especially for youth involved in crisis problems. Newspapers and radio and television programs developed a variety of I & R-type public media programs, including the popular "Call for Action" programs.

Expansion in the 1970s

Since the passage of the Older Americans Act Amendments of 1973, a major focus of the Administration on Aging (AOA) has been on the formation and development of a national network on aging. I & R has been a primary mechanism for linkages of services in state and local area agencies. One of the major contributions of AOA has been its support of extensive research projects on the evaluation and effectiveness of I & R services in age-integrated and age-segregated programs.

Spearheaded by AOA, a 15-member federal Interdepartmental Task Force was organized in 1974 to promote coordination of I & R networks with linkages to public and voluntary agencies on national, state, and local levels. AOA has, through working agreements with 15 federal agency representatives, promoted I & R training programs in accordance with guidelines formulated by the Interdepartmental Task Force.[2]

One of the member agencies of this Task Force, the U. S. Veterans Administration, has undertaken a national program of I & R training symposiums to instruct VA staff in I & R program development and to collaborate, where possible, with AOA agencies and other community agencies in I & R networks. The major participants in these symposiums have been social workers and Veterans Benefit Counselors from VA facilities.[3]

The designation of I & R as a social utility under Title XX legislation (1974) has been a major breakthrough in expanding I & R in concept and practice since it provides I & R services for all citizens irrespective of income, age, or residence. A growing number of states have already developed or are projecting I & R networks, either state-administered or under a "contract for services" with voluntary agencies.[4]

Interest in providing neighborhood information centers (NICs), which were built into the community action programs of the 1960s, increased in the 1970s. Consumer rights became more vocal: on the one hand, insisting upon access to personal social data and, on the other, demanding rights to confidentiality and privacy as reinforced by the Federal Privacy Act of 1974.

The public library has recently begun to emerge as a local community agency for I & R services. The capabilities of public libraries in providing I & R services were demonstrated in the Neighborhood Information Centers Projects conducted in five major cities under federal funding between 1972 and 1975. Librarians are increasingly assuming the responsibilities of human service intermediaries, which extend library services beyond the traditional reference files. New educational programs in I & R services have been developed in professional schools of library science as well as in inservice training programs for librarians. A new literature on I & R services is evolving in the library field, prompted by official recognition of I & R as a priority in "user-oriented services" by the American Library Association.[5]

Another notable development has been the organization of the National Alliance of Information and Referral Services (AIRS). Formally organized in 1972, AIRS has sought to develop standards, establish criteria, and promote communication and coordination among providers of I & R programs in public and voluntary sectors. As a major source for the dissemination of information on developments in I & R services, AIRS publishes a newsletter, a professional *I & R Quarterly,* a *Directory of I & R Agencies* and a *Directory of I & R Resources.* The national voluntary organizations of AIRS and the United Way of America have contributed significantly to the development of what has come to be an I & R movement.

In search of a model for an American I & R system, Alfred J. Kahn and his associates studied the British Citizens Advice Bureau and concluded that while the British Citizens Advice Bureaux (CABs) could not be wholly transposed to America, the I & R concept of a service modality to facilitate access should be initiated and instituted through experimentation and empirical experiences in the United States.[6] Concurrently, Zucker and Wittman also called attention to the CABs as I & R models for the improvement of access to services.[7, 8]

With the exception of Kahn, there is scanty reference to I & R operations in the professional social work literature. In 1971, Kahn described the state of the art of I & R services as "islands of experiments," and pointed to access services as a vehicle for redistribution and advocacy.[9] Addressing the field of public welfare in 1974, Kahn viewed the development of I & R services as a "beginning phase" in the overhauling of the American public welfare system. In recognition of the importance of I & R services, Kahn designated "Access Services" as a major category in the classification of all personal social services.[10]

Another national authority on I & R, Nicholas Long, developed a series of evaluative prescriptive studies on I & R programming. His classic article on "Information and Referral Services: A Brief History and Some Recommendations," documented the uneven development of I & R services in the public and voluntary sectors.[11]

Advances in information science and computer technology during the 1970s also promoted I & R programs. While manual I & R programs are still predominantly used, automated I & R services have spurred the rapid development of more elaborate and sophisticated I & R systems, capable of handling voluminous items of information with remarkable efficiency.[12]

Definition of I & R Services

Definitions of an I & R service vary enormously, depending on many factors including organizational setting, agency mission, available resources, and consumer characteristics. Although marked differences in I & R operations exist in the fields of health and social services, there is general agreement that an I & R service is essentially a *universal doorway to available resources, offered free of charge, and aimed to promote access for the inquirer and potential consumer. I & R services also serve as a vehicle for community planning through the utilization of its data-reporting system.* Thus I & R services are aimed to offer direct services in linking the consumer with an available appropriate and acceptable service and use the data for the purpose of health and social planning of agency services and community programs.

In order to make existing services more intelligible, accessible, and equitable for all citizens, I & R services have been organized to provide accurate, up-to-date information and then refer consumers to needed resources within a system that assures accountability. The application of I & R data for planning purposes is currently receiving increased attention in the community planning programs of health and social services.

The dual terms "information and referral" describe both a process and a product. As a process, it is inherent in all acts of human helping and cuts across all human service functions; as a product, I & R represents an organizational entity. Viewed as a process, most service providers in health and social agencies would agree that I & R services are inherent in all social helping processes and are variously incorporated in the formal intake process in social agencies.

As a product or entity, I & R services are distinguished from the usual services of direct service agencies. Criteria and standards have been formulated to arrive at an acceptable and recognized I & R organization. One of the earliest delineations of minimal organizational criteria was formulated by Bloksberg and Caso in their 1967 survey, which stipulated that an I & R service must be a formally organized service that provides I & R services as its primary task within an agency or subunit of the agency. The staff assigned to conduct the service is to consist of at least one part-time paid staff person. These criteria clearly emphasize the organizational structure of the I & R service.[13]

The first formal set of I & R standards developed by the United Way in 1973 regarded information and referral as both an organizational structure and as a task or function.[14] An expanded and updated version of the United Way standards and other earlier sets of standards was published by the Alliance of Information and Referral Services (AIRS) in 1978.[15] However, with no official enforcement or regulatory machinery, adherence to these standards remains an arbitrary choice. Nevertheless, the thrust is toward regulation and eventual accreditation of I & R services.

Service Dimensions

To date there is no clearly defined consensus on the specific functions of an I & R Service, nor is there absolute agreement on how these functions are to operate within an I & R program.

Kahn distinguishes between the *essential* components of information giving, advice, and referral from the *optional* components, which include counseling, advocacy outreach, consumer participation, and community planning. Concrete services, such as transportation and escort services, sometimes subsumed under outreach services, are also classified as optional.[16] Assuming a somewhat different approach, Long suggests that I

& R functions be added incrementally and in accordance with the readiness of agencies and staff to take on various functions appropriate for a particular agency at a particular time.[17]

It is generally helpful to view I & R functions as a spectrum of services which range on a continuum, from the simpler functions to the more complex in the provision of information, advice, referral, follow-up advocacy services, and provision for treatment if indicated. As noted on the following chart, multifaceted service roles are assigned to providers responsible for various I & R functions (see Figure 1). The six provider roles in Figure 1 reflect the broad range of responsibilities included within direct and indirect services in I & R programs. The information specialist, service intermediary and case advocate are involved with direct services; the class or policy advocate, administrator/planner and educator/trainer are relegated to indirect service functions. None of these roles is discrete or mutually exclusive, but rather occur in a combination or a blend of overlapping role-functions.

The *information specialist* is held accountable for the delivery of updated information on resources, generally organized within a resource file. Information-giving may entail "steering," which assumes that once the information is given the receiver or user of information is capable of proceeding without further assistance. Or it may involve "advice giving," which entails a process of helping the user to formulate a plan or a course of action.

For the *service intermediary,* the I & R task may involve brief counseling and/or referral to another agency based on an appropriate procedure of diagnostic assessment. Where the need for indepth counseling is indicated, either the service intermediary is so designated by the I & R agency or a referral is made to an appropriate agency for extended counseling, as diagnostically determined. Since referral procedures are usually not clearly defined or standardized, a decision regarding selective or universal follow-up generally reflects the agency's policy as well as the provider's judgment of the client's initiative and readiness to follow up on a referral. Long cautions against burdening the "already troubled client" by relying unduly on the client's motivation to follow through.[18] For such a client/patient, the need for advocacy is urgent.

The overall responsibility for program design, determination of program priorities, and for organizational decisions related to staff and agency budget is usually assumed by an *administrator/planner.* Evaluation of current I & R operations, assessment of priorities, and projections of new approaches in I & R service delivery generally fall within the major responsibilities assigned to the dual roles of the administrator/planner. These tasks may also entail community planning and service planning in collaboration with other formal and informal organizations.

Of equal importance to the direct service functions of I & R Services

Figure 1
Provider Roles for I & R Functions
In Direct and Indirect Services

		information giving (steering)
	Information Specialist	advice (for help in making plans)
		referral (for special information; for further services)
Direct Services		
		brief counseling (limited time)
	Service Intermediary	in-depth counseling (extended time)
		referral (for specialized service; for complex situations)
	Case Advocate	advocacy focused on assisting the individual consumer
		advocacy focused on service agency in behalf of individual and/or family
	Class (or Policy) Advocate	advocacy focused on aggregates of consumers
		advocacy focused on social action in behalf of a social cause
		agency planning
	Administrator/Planner	service planning
		community planning
Indirect Services		
		intra-agency program
	Educator/Trainer	inter-agency program
		inter-disciplinary program
		public education

are the capabilities of the I & R Reporting System to serve as a valuable data base for the planning of health and social services. Increased attention is being given to I & R as a mechanism for health and social planning, based on the capability of I & R service statistics to reveal gaps, inadequacies, duplications, and insufficiencies of services. I & R data also reflect consumer characteristics, the incidence and severity of reported social problems, and the aggregate demand for services.[19]

In an era of increased emphasis on mandated planning in the field of health (Health Systems Agencies) and social welfare (Title XX—Comprehensive Annual Services Program Plan), an I & R system is a significant data source which can reflect needs assessment, service utilization, geographic distribution of population, and resource inventories. The extent to which the planning and research components of an I & R program can be carried out often depends upon the level of sophistication of staff and operation of educational training programs.[20]

Training and educational programs may be the responsibility of the administration, but may also be carried out by professional consultants, assigned intra-agency staff members or by prearranged interagency collaborative training programs. A variety of educational and training programs for I & R providers has been developed by professional schools and social agencies to meet the widely divergent interests of multidisciplinary providers and various levels of staff, including paraprofessionals and volunteers.

The *educator/trainer* is generally responsible for two types of educational programs: attention to the organization and delivery of health and social services, including knowledge of regulations, procedures, and current and projected legislation; and emphasis on skills in interviewing, counseling, and other interpersonal helping skills.

To prepare professionals with expertise in I & R program development and service delivery, the Adelphi University School of Social Work since 1975 has developed an I & R training and research program for undergraduate, graduate, and doctoral social work students. Under the sponsorship of the Social Policy Center within the School of Social Work, the I & R program has focused on program development in field instruction settings. The center also offers inservice training programs for I & R agency staff as well as interdisciplinary workshops. Utilization of students in the training and supervision of volunteers in I & R programs has been of particular interest to I & R agencies.

Graduate schools of library science have also developed special curriculums for instruction in I & R expertise, including field internships and research projects. For example, the University of Toledo, Ohio, has offered a Community Information Specialist Course for library students, which incorporates I & R program development skills for professional librarians. At Columbia University a joint program in I & R Services is offered to students in the School of Social Work by faculty members from the School of Library Science. A promising trend is the recognition of the advisability of greater collaboration among professional providers of I & R Services.[21]

Organizational Dimensions

Differences in I & R services vary enormously depending on whether the agency is the hot line of a free-standing storefront service or whether it is ancillary to other primary services, such as the I & R office in the local public health department or local library. The kinds of I & R services offered will depend on whether the I & R service is located in an urban neighborhood vicinity, a suburban shopping area, or a sparsely populated rural area.

I & R services are most often conducted by telephone, particularly for hot line assistance and public information inquiries. However, I & R services are also provided as walk-in services, usually a preferred entry for services by the elderly. I & R services can also be conducted by correspondence, particularly when the I & R location is at a distance from the consumer.

In view of the vast organizational and structural differences among I & R agencies, the services provided vary significantly in quality, substance, and outcome. Experience with I & R programs indicates that a public relations program is necessary to create consumer awareness of this community service. The use of mass media, including wide dissemination of publications and personal contacts, is vital in informing the public of the availability of I & R services. Underutilized I & R programs without an effective public relations program, need to be prepared to meet the demands of consumers when extensive publicity campaigns are conducted.

A primary determinant of an I & R service is the organizational auspices under which the service operates: a legally constituted nonprofit corporate entity, a function of such a legally constituted corporate entity, or a function of a federal, state, or local governmental agency. A growing trend is for agencies to collaborate through a service network in which I & R provides the service entry for information and referral purposes.

In most comprehensive I & R agencies, funding is usually received from multiple sources. A major source is federal Title XX funds channeled through Title XX state allocations programs. Local communities also use varied innovative approaches for funding, including private foundations, utility companies, industrial establishments, and local governmental agencies. In-kind provisions for the operations of I & R services offered by public libraries, planning councils, and other local resources are also significant sources.

Although the base of an I & R system generally requires a centralized operation, the delivery of I & R services is primarily a local function. Interest in locality-based services, with a focus on "back to the old neighborhood," which evolved in the 1960s, became even more vital in the 1970s with the continuing impact of consumerism and demands for accountability.[22] In response to these pressures, the public library, took on the responsibility of I & R services. Libraries now offer information on human services to local citizens, who may not necessarily be book-borrowing patrons. Bringing the service as close to the consumer as possible is the thrust of an I & R agency.

Outposts for I & R programs continue to emerge at focal points in the community where people tend to congregate and seek out services, that is, neighborhood schools, train depots and bus stations, stores and shopping plazas, post office branches, and local banks. Where distance to services is a problem, I & R mobile units are used.

In making choices, agencies are faced with major organizational decisions in the development of the centralized base of an information system and the operation of a decentralized service unit within a service network.

The history of I & R services in the United States reflects a tendency toward more specialized, rather than general services. Since the programs in the early 1960s required professional social workers, greater specialization resulted. Experience in community programs organized under the auspices of the Administration on Aging (AOA) generally reflects a trend to expand from age-segregated to age-integrated I & R programs, that is, from a more specialized program to a more general program. While it is generally conceded that I & R services should ideally operate as an autonomous service, free of organizational and professional biases, specialized health and mental health I & R services provided by host agencies are more predominant than the free-standing model.

How to provide a general unbiased portal of entry to health and social services, which also incorporates specific information on particular health disorders or generic groups of disorders, remains a challenge for future service planners and policy makers.

Given the multidiscipline and multilevels of staff in I & R programs, including professionals, paraprofessionals, and volunteers the responsibility of meeting the infinite needs of *all* citizens in a program that maintains a universal entry to services appears awesome. The organizational decision of "who does what" in an I & R service is often defined by the mission and tradition of the agency as well as by organizational resources and consumer expectation.

A significant consequence of the locality-based community action programs of the 1960s was the blending of consumer-provider roles. This duality of roles equipped the volunteer and the new paraprofessional with keen understanding of the problems of local residents in reaching care. It also reflected the demands of consumerism for access to services through self-help and local volunteer activities. In I & R services, volunteers have traditionally taken on the major tasks of core staff as well as ancillary service tasks.

In the I & R programs designed for specialized health and mental health agencies in the early 1960s the professional social worker was specified as the mandated provider, particularly in the fields of the handicapped and the emotionally disturbed. However, I & R services are not the domain of any one profession. While social workers tend to occupy managerial positions in I & R programs, nurses, teachers, librarians, psychologists, and many other professionals are also involved in I & R service delivery, including a recent infusion of computer specialists.

The I & R literature questions whether the professional is absolutely essential to the effective delivery of I & R programs. Some authorities maintain that professionals have had a restrictive rather than a promotional effect on I & R development.[23] The general consensus is that a mix of staff members, including professionals, paraprofessionals, and volunteers, is desirable. However, which tasks for what level of staff still remain unspecified and untested.[24]

Operational Dimensions

An indispensable operational tool of an I & R system is the maintenance of a reliable and updated resource file, organized with cross-references by listings of agencies or organizations, services or problems, and geographic area. Agency files usually include such data as hours and days of services, eligibility criteria, intake procedures, waiting lists, and descriptions of agency programs.

The underpinning of an I & R service is the *information system,* which provides selected and systematized data on resources to meet human service needs and are available for health and social planning. A review of the current state of this art in I & R programs reveals an impressive development of growing numbers of sophisticated manual and computerized I & R systems which aim to standardize information on human services and consumer service statistics.

To date, information systems have been designed primarily for the *service provider.* With the advent of the computer, providers in social agencies have established information systems on consumer data as valuable tools for client-tracking and case management, especially for quality control, cost effectiveness, and service efficiency. While the technology of management information systems in social agencies has continued to advance for the service provider, overwhelming barriers to services persist for the consumer.

In the health field, we are involved with perhaps the most highly developed technological human information service systems that are capable of systematizing and monitoring patient care programs, medical progress reports, hospital discharge data, and the storage, refinement, and retrieval of vast amounts of medical and social data. An impressive development of computerized health information systems has occurred during the past decade which deals with aggregated health data monitored over extended periods of time.

In the medical field, patient data are recorded to account for primary care, document medical care information for eligibility for third-party payments, and report on personal health data as required by various social service programs such as those in public welfare, employment, and rehabilitation.[25]

In the health field, it is essential to distinguish between medical information systems, hospital information systems, and health information systems. Medical information systems are designed for the recording of patient information and patient tracking. Hospital information systems operate primarily to expedite organizational management and to establish fiscal accountability for services extended within the facility. Unlike either of the above, health information systems operate as systematized funds of data for information on total populations, gathered at regular intervals to record vital statistics and epidemiological phenomena within designated time periods.

Little organized attempt has been made to combine medical data with community resource information in patient planning, discharge, and follow-up. To what extent the Problem Oriented Record (POR) can be used in linking the patient/consumer to an appropriate community resource has been minimally explored. Essentially, POR is an administrative tool used for patient accountability based on problem identification and the development of a plan related to each identified problem. The potential for combining health and social services information into an integrated human resources system has yet to be demonstrated.

While there is no single I & R system model that effectively links health and social services in a unified system, various approaches have been used in I & R programs to span the areas of health and social services. Three broad categories of information systems which include examples of I & R programs related to health and social services are: interagency programs, intra-agency programs, and health information systems.

One example of an *interagency program* is the United Way Services Identification System (UWASIS classification system) based on major goals and subgoals for human services. Optimal health is defined as a goal in the attainment of "an optimal level of wellness" for all individuals, whereby service systems are thus geared to the promotion and maintenance of health, treatment, and, where feasible, cure of disease and rehabilitation of the handicapped. UWASIS has provided the base for numerous adaptations of I & R systems, including the highly developed systems in Louisville, Kentucky, and Hampton Roads, Virginia.[26]

Another is the SEARCH program, developed at the University of Southern California Medical School, Los Angeles, that identified resources according to correlated matrices of health problems and social service resources.[27] And a third is the WIS program in Wisconsin based on the SEARCH model. It is an I & R network of heterogeneous health and social service agencies.[28]

Intra-Agency Programs are represented by a patient representative programs and discharge referral systems. Many large hospitals as well as some public mental hospitals and Health Maintenance Organizations have appointed patient representatives (PR), either as paid staff or volunteers. A major function of a patient representative is to understand the complexities of the health care establishment and identify policies and procedures that result in misunderstanding, hardship, or poor service. To carry patient representative functions, I & R services are either maintained within the PR program or sought out by connecting with another source for I & R services.

An intra-agency I & R-type advocacy system has been developed at The Mount Sinai Hospital in New York City. Patient representatives operate as ombudsmen and are accountable to the administration of the social service department. A system of designated social work staff members for specific information on selected resources has also been incorporated in this intra-agency I & R-type system.[29]

Experience with internal I & R systems has shown benefits to providers as well as consumers in monitoring the route of patients/consumers through the complex maze of health care service units, departments, and facilities. In addition, the intra-agency I & R service experience has resulted in increased levels of effectiveness in service delivery as reported by hospital administrators and as reflected in consumer responses.

A computer assisted discharge referral system, identified as CINCH, is designed to match its resource data profiles with patient data profiles at discharge to assist providers in appropriate referrals to community resources.[30]

Health information systems can be provider focused or consumer focused. A public information approach is used by the Information & Referral Manual System (IRMA) of New York City which has, through computerized classifications of resources, produced specialized directories of health and social services organizations. IRMA currently serves as the

I & R system for the Human Resources Administration of the New York City Department of Social Services.[31]

A consumer-focused service in the medical care field is TEL-MED which has, since 1972, developed a general medical information system for the public in over one hundred cities in the United States. TEL-MED has been combined with the Community Council Information System in Rhode Island, whereby the caller is directed to further assistance by referral to a designated social worker, available at the consumer's choice.[32]

To what extent can we collaborate, link up, or amalgamate these information systems to create greater access to comprehensive health care services? Should health consumer information systems and general I & R programs continue to develop independently or can we collaborate in our efforts toward a joint information system in the fields of health and social services?

Assessments and Projections

I & R services undoubtedly will continue to expand as tight budgets and consumer demands for accountability point to the advisability of maximum utilization of existing resources. The recognition of I & R as a universal service modality under Title XX legislation, and the trend toward intergovernmental collaboration and interagency alliances in I & R programs, indicate an increased growth potential for such programs. Sophisticated automated technology in I & R management suggests vast opportunities for unprecedented growth.

One of the costs of rapid, unplanned growth has been the proliferation of I & R services in many health and social service agencies. A 1978 study conducted by the U. S. General Accounting Office (GAO) concluded that consolidation of I & R activities is essential and that comprehensive I & R services should be promoted. Describing current I & R Services as a "complex system that should be improved," the GAO noted that "the orderless growth has resulted in a specialized, fragmented system characterized by . . . duplication of and competition between services and functions . . . waste of resources . . . barriers obstructing access . . . and inadequate services."[33] Furthermore, the GAO study found that I & R centers established to consolidate activities and provide comprehensive services were competing with other providers for clientele and appropriations.

In view of the lack of a national policy and plan for I & R, the GAO report proposed "a single Federal focal point with the responsibility and authority for coordinating Federal programs for community-based information and referral services."[34] Upon reviewing the recommendations of the GAO report, the Inspector General of the Department of HEW took issue on a "broad brush approach" to I & R activities, and suggested that some differentiation should be made between a general information service and specialized I & R services. Furthermore, HEW maintained "that coordination and consolidation of I & R will not be sufficient without a basic reorganization of human service systems."[35]

While I & R programs may facilitate access, I & R cannot make up for the gaps and inadequacies of existing health and social programs, nor can it solve the broader societal problems of mass unemployment, poverty, and discrimination. Problems of confidentiality and selectivity of information remain undefined and in need of policy formulation. And although I & R services are, by definition, free of charge to the consumer, the costs of operation may entail sizeable investment. On a cautious note, I & R services need to guard against developing the very bureaucratic rigidities they seek to overcome.

Policy Implications

The universal concern for health, which transcends age, income, or race, logically fits into the universal open door policy of an I & R service. While the goal of equal health status may be unrealistic, greater accessibility to health services through I & R services can bring about greater equity. Kahn highlights the redistributive potential in access services, which is capable of bringing "more services to more people."[36]

I & R may also promote "better health for more people" through an information access system that responds to consumer/patient inquiries and monitors the user through the maze of health and social services within the health and medical setting as well as in the community. Informal health consumer groups, such as self-care, self-help and share-care groups, which represent important avenues for health maintenance, are often in search of reliable information sources for access to existing services. In a sense, an I & R service is a vehicle for community health education; in practice, health education is a product of a comprehensive I & R service.

Prevention can be promoted through an I & R service by providing systematic access to a service and follow through, either before the problem occurs (primary prevention) or by arresting or ameliorating the effects of a problem (secondary prevention) or by assisting with the effective treatment of an existing condition (tertiary prevention). While logic supports the assumption of preventive intervention through an access system, the efficacy of prevention through the modality of more integrated and coherent I & R services is an untapped area for research.[37]

Increased recognition of I & R services as a data base for health and social planning is more evident as agencies and communities seek more rational bases for assessment of needs and resources. The lack of effective planning in the reentry of discharged mental patients into the community has clearly pointed to the need for locally operated I & R systems which can link primary health care and community health care, facility-care and home-care, and acute care services and chronic health care programs.

A significant first step of an I & R service is to link up with existing I & R programs wherever available and feasible. Local I & R services will vary according to the socioeconomic conditions prevalent in the community and in accord with the local population. Commonalities and differences in urban, suburban, and rural I & R systems will need to be considered. Certain population target groups require special consideration: the growing proportion of elderly in the total population, the expanding numbers of deinstitutionalized mental patients, and the multifaceted concerns of the chronically ill. While specialized services are required for the particular needs of designated target groups, linkages need to be established with formally organized social service agencies and with those support systems in the community which function as informal human helping networks, including the primary family, extended families, friendship groups, fraternal organizations, and block groups. I & R services are viewed as vehicles for the promotion of linkages which extend beyond single service parameters and organizational boundaries.

Rather than adding a super-structure of I & R services to the already unwieldy health care system, an incremental approach toward planned linkages of existing human resources is proposed in preference to large scale reform. A review of the developments in I & R programs and in health information systems suggests the advisability, expediency, and economy of an integrated human resources information system that can link a consumer to needed resources through intra-agency and interagency networks. This broad-based community approach transcends the physical boundaries and confines of medical and social agency facilities, including hospitals. It places the health institution as a major hub in a community network of other service outlets to guide and monitor a consumer's route "in and out" of the health and social services network. This viable approach to an I & R network must take into account the nonmedical as well as the medical setting, the public library as well as the hospital, the social agency as well as the health clinic, the priest as well as the doctor.

Research and empirical studies of I & R operations will suggest further capabilities for facilitating access and helping persons to reach needed health care and social services.

References

1. Richard M. Titmuss. "Welfare State and Welfare Society," Chapter XI, in *Commitment to Welfare.* New York: Pantheon Books, 1968, pp. 124–137.

2. U.S. Department of Health, Education and Welfare, Administration on Aging, Office of Human Development Services. *Report of the Interdepartmental Task Force on Information and Referral.* Washington, D.C., September 1978. DHEW Pub. No. (OHDS) 79-20045.

3. Risha W. Levinson. "Programs of Information and Referral Services: U.S. Veterans Administration, Findings and Recommendations," Unpublished Preliminary Report, July 31, 1978.

4. Jerrold Hercenberg. "Information and Referral Services Funding Under Title XX." In *Proceedings of the Information and Referral Roundtable, 1976,* Alliance of Information and Referral Services, pp. 61–65.

5. Dorothy Turick. *Community Information Services in Libraries, Library Journal,* Sherral Report, No. 5, November 1977; also see Clara S. Jones, ed., *Public Library Information and Referral Service.* Syracuse, N.Y.: Gaylord Bros., Inc., 1978.

6. Alfred J. Kahn. *Neighborhood Information Centers: A Study and Some Proposals.* New York: Columbia University School of Social Work, 1966.

7. Mildred Zucker. "Citizens Advice Bureaus: The Better Way," *Social Work* 10:4:85–91, Oct. 1965.

8. Milton Wittman. "The Feasibility of Citizens' Advice Bureaux in American Social Services," London, England: Unpublished Manuscript, March 1966.

9. Alfred J. Kahn. "Perspectives on Access to Social Services," *Social Work* 15:2:96–97, April 1970.

10. Alfred J. Kahn. *Social Policy and Social Services.* 2nd edition, New York, Random House, 1979, pp. 26–31.

11. Nicholas Long. "Information and Referral Services: A Short History and Some Recommendations," *Social Service Review* 47:1:49–62, March 1973.

12. Allvin L. Sallee. "Evaluation Methodology for Information and Referral." In *Proceedings of the Information and Referral Roundtable,* Alliance of the Information and Referral Services, May 1977.

13. Leonard M. Bloksberg and Elizabeth K. Caso. *Survey of Information and Referral Services Existing Within the United States: Final Report.* Waltham, Mass., Brandeis University, Florence Heller Graduate School for Advanced Studies in Social Welfare, 1967, p. 62.

14. United Way of America. *National Standards for Information and Referral Services.* Alexandria, Virginia, United Way, 1973, pp. 1–16.

15. Alliance of Information and Referral Services, Inc. *National Standards for Information and Referral Services.* Phoenix, Arizona, International Graphics Co., May 21, 1978.

16. Kahn. *Social Policy and Social Services. Op. cit.,* pp. 166–167.

17. Nicholas Long. *Resource File, Information Giving, Referral and Follow Through, Escort and Outreach.* Interstudy Associates, Minneapolis, Minnesota, 1972–1975.

18. Nicholas Long *et al. Information and Referral Centers: A Functional Analysis.* Minneapolis, Minnesota, American Rehabilitation Foundation, 1971, p. 14.

19. Shirley Zimmerman and Richard Sterne. "The Use of Information and Referral Service Data in Social Planning and Administration." Paper presented at the Fifth NASW Professional Symposium, San Diego, California, November 1977. (Unpublished manuscript.)

20. Ronald E. Hansen. "One Classification System for Information and Referral and for Planning." Presented at Roundtable Meeting of AIRS, National Conference on Social Welfare, Annual Meeting, 1978, Los Angeles, California.

21. Miriam Braverman and Miles Martin. "The Education of Information and Referral Librarians and Implications for the Future." In *Public Library Information and Referral Service,* ed. by Clara S. Jones, *Op. cit.,* pp. 139–153; also see Risha W. Levinson, "Professional Partners in Local Information and Referral Services: Librarians and Social Workers." Position Paper presented at the I & R Institute for Professional Librarians: The Public Library as Community Information Center, sponsored by C. W. Post College and Nassau Library System, June 2, 1975. (Unpublished.)

22. Joseph L. Vigilante. "Back to the Old Neighborhood." *Social Service Review* 50:2:202, June 1976.

23. Nicholas Long. "Information and Referral Services in the 1980's: Where Should They Go? Who Should Lead? Will Anyone Follow?" Information and Referral: *The Journal of the Alliance of Information and Referral Systems* 1:1:16–17, Spring 1979.

24. Risha W. Levinson. "Training/Technology/Manpower: Information and Referral to the 21st Century." Proceedings of the Information and Referral Roundtable, Washington, D.C., 1976, pp. 21–32.

25. Alan F. Westin. *Computers, Health Records, and Citizens' Rights,* Washington, D.C., U.S. Department of Commerce, December 1976, pp. 8–11.

26. United Way of America. *UWASIS and Its Uses,* Alexandria, Virginia: United Way of America, 1975; also see *UWASIS II: A Taxonomy of Social Goals and Human Service Programs.* Alexandria, Virginia: United Way of America, 1976.

27. Joy Cauffman. *Inventory of Human Services: Medical and Social.* Los Angeles, California, University of Southern California School of Medicine, 1972, 3rd edition.

28. Nicholas Long and Leslie Yonce. *Information and Referral Services: Evaluation Design for a Network Demonstration.* Minneapolis, Minnesota, Interstudy, February 1974.

29. Ruth Ravich and Helen Rehr. "Ombudsman Program Provides Feedback." *Hospitals* 48:18:63–67, Sept. 16, 1974.

30. Benjamin Papell and Annemarie F. Crocetti. *"CINCH:* A Model of Practice for Community Health." Oxford, England: Symposium on Community Health Information Systems, September 5–8, 1972, pp. 1–24.

31. Rae Brooks and Daniel J. Eastman. *IRMA: A Computer-Assisted Citizen Information Resource System,* Volumes I and II. New York, Administration and Management Research Association of New York City, Inc., 1974.

32. Teletronics Information Systems. Redlands, California, United Recording Electronics Industry (undated); Tel-Med Program for Rhode Island. Providence, Rhode Island, Council for Community Services, Inc., November 1974.

33. *Information and Referral for People Needing Services: A Complex System That Should be Improved.* Washington, D.C., Comptroller General of the United States, March 20, 1978, p. i.

34. *Ibid.* p. iii.

35. *Ibid.* p. 51 (Appendix IX).

36. Kahn. "Perspectives on Access to Social Services," *Op. cit.,* p. 96.

37. Risha W. Levinson. "Gateways to Prevention: Access Service Systems." Invitational Paper. Council on Social Work Education, Annual Program Meeting, New Orleans, Louisiana, February 27, 1978. (Unpublished.)

Chapter IV

Community Health Ombudsman

HELEN HABERMAN DEITCH

Consumers and providers of health and medical care interact in a number of complex ways to determine the nature and quality of services. Political decisions are made about the allocation of resources for the health sector. These decisions are affected by the overlapping interests of provider and consumer groups as well as those of the general public. Each group has different sources and degrees of power in policy formation and derives differential benefits. While they may form coalitions in seeking certain legislation, they are often competitive with each other. To a large degree, the extent and way in which health and medical services are provided is determined by resolution of the differences between the interest groups, which is then embodied in federal legislation and policy.[1]

While health and medical care services are greatly influenced by federal policy, providers and consumers are engaged in decision-making at regional, institutional, and personal levels, and these affect the nature and quality of care in a more immediate way. Physicians and their professional organizations still largely control the medical care system even though there has been a trend toward increased pluralism. At best, the loosening of power has not led to an equal partnership between physicians and consumers. Rather, as Navarro and others have suggested, the control of the health care system is moving toward an oligarchy in which physicians share control with hospital boards of trustees and administrators, large corporate drug and medical supply company executives, and governmental officials, all of whom have overlapping reference groups oriented to the interests of the upper middle class.[2] Consumers, especially those belonging to marginal economic groups and minorities, continue to compete relatively unsuccessfully for an opportunity to influence medical care services.

Despite changes in the health care system, society still places great value on the relationship between patient and physician. However, as health care has become more bureaucratized and the relationship between physician and patient less personal, more formal controls have augmented earlier reliance on ethical standards and personal obligations to protect both of them. State and local governments, through their regulatory agencies, inspect, audit, and use fiscal incentives and penalties to try to set standards and enforce the quality of medical care. They are increasingly requiring that physicians monitor their own activities through such mechanisms as peer review organizations. These efforts have been only partially effective, and the individual patient/consumer continues to experience unevenness in the quality of care received. The patient/consumer also has difficulty in gaining access to or receptivity by state and local regulatory agencies which are entrusted with monitoring the quality of care. Informal and formal intermediary mechanisms have developed to increase the capacity of individual citizens to make complaints about unmet needs, evaluate the quality of care provided, and redress grievance when the services offered are insufficient or of poor quality.

Ombudsmen and Advocates

Ombudsmen have had an established role in a number of western nations for several centuries. They are a reflection of a recognized need of citizens for protection against the misuse of power by appointed or elected officials. Some system was needed to make sure that judges, civil servants, and military officers in their enforcement of the law did not do damage to individual rights or benefits. The ombudsman system has been adopted in 14 countries throughout the world. Today, even small developing nations like Mauritius and Guyana have national ombudsmen. While they may have different capacities to initiate investigations, greater or lesser power in influencing change, and a broader or narrower scope of intervention, they are similar in major intent and function.

What, exactly, are government ombudsmen? What are they expected to do? Walter Gelhorn identifies an ombudsman as one force in a network of mechanisms that limit and regulate government bureaucracy and seek to protect citizens from official injustice.[3] While legislatures, the courts, and special regulatory agencies are the most basic means of holding bureaucrats accountable, and present a "before the fact" approach in that they set down laws and standards for equitable treatment of the total population, an ombudsman essentially operates "after the fact," investigating complaints of individuals and attempting to bring about a redress of grievances when necessary.[4] Ombudsmen are, in essence, adjudicators of injustices created by the inequities or misapplication of laws and administrative regulations. They act as a mechanism for receiving citizen complaints and as a means of redress of grievance. They are not expected to reform basic political structures or to solve large-scale social or economic problems. Rather, they are concerned with the effect of administrative behavior and decision-making on individual citizens. Characteristically, ombudsmen possess personal prestige as independent, nonpolitical, impartial individuals with a high value on fairness. They are usually sponsored by an organization or legislative body outside of the system they investigate in order to ensure objectivity and protect them from bureaucratic pressures. They are visible and accessible to anyone who wishes to make a complaint.[5]

In most places an ombudsman is appointed by an arm of government. He may serve alone or with a staff for a fixed term or until retirement. He has the right of subpoena to investigate complaints or grievances of any citizen. Since he has authority only to make recommendations, his powers are quite limited. His effectiveness derives from his prestige, his capacity to move freely in the administrative system, and from the reporting and publicizing of his findings. He cannot override substantive decisions of judges or other public officials. He does not handle grievances against private companies or private individuals. Not every inquiry received by an ombudsman requires investigation. He screens complaints as, in some cases, only information is required, while in others, advice is provided about existing resources and government agencies to which the citizen may apply for assistance.

Sweden has the oldest classic ombudsman program, now almost 200 years old. It has served as a model for subsequent programs established elsewhere. Sweden's Parliament appoints the ombudsman and provides funds for operating the program. The ombudsman serves for a four-year term, which has occasionally been extended by reappointment for as long as 16 years. Usually the deputy moves into the top spot when it is vacated.

All complaints from the public must be in writing. Many complaints do not warrant extensive investigation and can be handled informally. Many others are referred to the proper agency for handling. Ombudsmen have full discretion to decide which cases will be investigated. In addition to reviewing individual cases they make "roving inspections" of government agencies, writing ahead to the administrator to announce the visit. Ombudsmen may examine the agency's reports and records and, if there is evidence of maladministration, may initiate a written inquiry or, in serious cases, hold public hearings. The responsible government official always has a right to a hearing. Cooperation of agency administrators is considered crucial. The ombudsman makes sure he is not regarded as someone whom the administrator should keep out. In practice, he usually enjoys the confidence of both citizens and administrators.

Often in response to similar complaints from more than one individual, as well as from public press reports of abuse of individuals, the ombudsman conducts longer-term investigations and makes public recommendations. Parliament does not have the right to control these investigations or recommendations, but can respond to them in a purely advisory manner. A standing committee of the Parliament spot checks the ombudsman's reports and may submit questions to him or request an opinion for parliamentary debate.

Since the ombudsman system has been operating for such a long time, Sweden does not have to promote the ombudsman service. Of 3,577 new cases registered in 1972, the service dealt with the majority (76%) before the end of the year. Ten percent of the complaints concerned medical care delivery.

Community-Based Health Ombudsman and Advocacy Programs

It is only in the last decade that community-based ombudsman and advocate programs have been established to deal with specific grievances about the functioning of the health system. The British system, founded in 1973, is perhaps the best known. It was the first ombudsman program where health services were separated from other government ombudsmen services. Under the National Health Service Reorganization Act (1973), a Health Services Commissioner, appointed by the Queen, heads a staff of 20 ombudsmen for England and 2 each for Scotland and Wales.

Since the role of British ombudsmen lies in protecting citizens in a broad range of health matters, complaints may relate to patient care, professional behavior, misconduct, or failure in communication and administrative procedures. For example, in maternity units, a patient may object to the inconvenience of an overly long waiting period before admission. In mental hospitals complaints tend to center around refusal to admit a patient, assaults by staff, pressure on patients to have electroconvulsive therapy and complaints from the family after a suicide. In homes for geriatric patients, unkind treatment may be cited. The ombudsmen also handle many cases resulting from failure in communication and the negligence of administrators in handling patients' direct complaints.

Any member of the public or someone acting on his behalf may complain to the Commissioner or a staff member. Members of Parliament may forward complaints they receive on health matters to the Commissioner. The complaint must be directed against a "relevant body," a regional area or special health authority. Written reports of all cases and their disposition are submitted to Parliament quarterly.

The Health Services Commissioner (ombudsman) "borrows" his staff for three to five years from the National Health Service and from other civil services, returning them after that time to their regular positions. This is in line with the British policy of developing a flexible civil service with health professionals capable of shifting functions. Staff may come from any discipline, but the Commissioner has traditionally been a former hospital administrator.

How does Britain limit the powers of the commissioner? 1. He cannot make clinical judgments about the way a doctor practices medicine. The medical profession has maintained protection and jurisdiction over this area of practice. Complaints against physicians go to a family practitioner committee, others to a health laboratory service board when appropriate. However, if a patient complaints about a procedural matter or about the way service is provided, such as the way a family practitioner committee handles a request for a change of doctor or deals with medical records, the ombudsman can investigate it. 2. He cannot deal with problems of staff personnel. 3. He cannot direct an authority to act nor can he start legal proceedings. 4. He has no power to make financial restitution. Affirmatively, the commissioner has power to bring an unresolved problem to the attention of a higher authority for action. He is not forced to rely solely on his persuasive powers at that level, but may go to Parliament with his case. He may also counsel complainants to seek legal advice.

The prerogatives of the ombudsman have been consistently resisted by the medical profession in Great Britain, and were only reluctantly accepted in a limited form after a series of public inquiries into scandals over abuse of patients by the staffs of several psychiatric and geriatric hospitals. While an ombudsman has authority to receive complaints about the organization of hospitals and clinics, the clinical autonomy of the physician is still held to be sacrosanct and not open to investigation. An ongoing problem is that the ombudsman service is staffed by health professionals of various disciplines on loan from the same organizational establishment they then seek to investigate, and there is some question about their capacity to be unbiased and to be accountable to consumers. The Health Services Commissioner, traditionally a former hospital administrator, has methods of approaching problems and a value system that tends to be derived from his own reference group. Another difficulty with the program emanates from the traditional British value on written reports. All complaints from consumers must be in writing. This puts a burden on those consumers with limited education or skill in writing and tends to deter them from making complaints.[6]

A recent study of the British system made by the U. S. Department of Health, Education and Welfare (now Department of Health and Human Services) recommended that the British experience should be considered if a National Health System is established in this country.[7] Meanwhile, the need for an impartial outside service to help solve patient problems in the United States has been felt by many different kinds of

organizations, groups, and institutions. Ombudsmen or advocacy programs are being established in the United States at state, city and local
levels under a variety of auspices.

While the ombudsman system is characterized as objective, unbiased,
independent, and impartial, the advocate system is considered as a parti-
san of the group it represents. An advocate's efforts are applied exclusively
in service of the client's interests and no claims are made to neutrality.[8]
The ideological approach of advocacy is that there are individuals and
groups who have been disadvantaged by prejudice and injustice and are
relatively powerless in their relations with social institutions. They need
active intercession and support to gain access to services and entitlements
from which they may be barred. The implication of the advocacy concept
is that social institutions, at least in part, have caused and maintained the
disadvantaged in that status and that pressure toward institutional change
is required in order to improve services to them. Advocates support and
advise their clients as well as represent them in their dealings with administrative officials and agencies. They apply their special knowledge and
skill to help an individual or group to develop a countervailing force to
powerful organizations.

The advocacy concept was borrowed from the legal model, and just
as a lawyer furthers a client's interests by the use of a variety of strategies,
an advocate for a community group can apply a range of tactics. Depending on an assessment of the situation and the goals to be achieved, an
advocate may employ such collaborative techniques as obtaining information, educating, problem-solving, engaging in joint action, and various
forms of persuasion. When differences between the community group and
the institution are great, more coercive techniques, such as maneuvering,
bargaining, and negotiation may be used. Openly adversary techniques—
protests, demonstrations, boycotts, and other disruptions—are used only
when there is marked dissension.[9]

An example of a community based advocacy program is the Health
Policy Advisory Center (Health-PAC). Its establishment was precipitated
by a variety of exposés of abuses in the health system in New York City
in the mid-and late-1960's. At first, Health-PAC's purpose was to conduct
research and analyze health policy. Later it expanded its service to include
monitoring, educational activities, and providing technical assistance to
other community groups attempting to improve health services for themselves. In contrast to the British ombudsman and many Office of Economic Opportunity (federal) programs, Health-PAC has no official sanction or powers. In this status lie both its advantages and disadvantages.
Privately funded, it has relative independence to investigate and analyze
all aspects of health services and to publicize its findings. Its preferred
stance is adversarial since it perceives the health industry as a vast medi-
cal-industrial complex, inimical to the interests of patient/consumers,

more interested in consolidating control over health resources than in providing service.

Health-PAC has taken advocacy positions in relation to the public municipal hospitals in New York City, challenging the concept of affiliation with voluntary hospitals and raising questions about fiscal accountability. It has also taken strong positions for setting occupational safety standards in hospitals, for safeguarding the rights of women and prisoners in relation to health services, and has offered training sessions for Community Advisory Board members to help them exert more influence in municipal hospitals. Its style is informal in order to facilitate access to community groups. It requires no formal written requests and attempts to provide expert information and technical assistance of immediate usefulness to health activists. Its effectiveness is in the use of exposés to stimulate public awareness to health issues and in supporting radical movements toward change in the health system. Private funding has supported the capacity of this organization to take an adversary stance, but insufficient funds to consistently maintain its activities have also limited its effectiveness.

Self-Help Groups

Mutual help groups or self-help organizations are another form of a community-based program that attempts to affect and evaluate the quality of health care. By definition, a mutual self-help group limits its membership to those who have common problems and who expect to offer each other help, guidance, and support in dealing with those problems. In contrast to health advocacy organizations like Health-PAC, it draws largely on the resources and the experiences of its membership in pursuing its program. Control of the organization is maintained by its members who are both providers and consumers of its services, and who have no special expertise except that which has been generated by trial and error experiences with their common problems. The services of professionals are sometimes employed, but they do not control the policy of the group.

Self-help organizations can be classified by their primary function: fund-raising; political action, which includes changing laws and regulations and affecting public attitudes; personal help; and consumer advocacy. Health organizations of all four types are common and their relationships with the medical care system range from supportive to oppositional.

Grass roots self-help organizations with an advocacy and monitoring stance in relation to health problems are becoming increasingly common all over the United States. For example, in 1970 and 1971 a group of parents started the Benevolent Society for Retarded Children in New York City as a section of the state parent program. The efforts of this group were abetted by the Women's Organization for Retarded Children

(WORC), another self-appointed group that did friendly visiting at Willowbrook, a 6,000-bed institution for the mentally retarded in New York City. They organized protests against conditions there, and raised funds that eventually helped finance a legal case against the institution.

These self-selected advocates for the mentally retarded achieved many of their goals. A Federal court imposed standards to be met by the institution and appointed a review panel to monitor the process. A majority of the former residents of the institution now live in the community instead of in the institution and conditions have improved for those who remain.

While the membership of the WORC and other such groups is composed of families of patients, other community-based self-help groups are made up of patients themselves. Increasingly, former mental patients have banded together to help other patients still in hospitals and those just released who need assistance in finding homes and jobs. One of the most interesting of these self-help groups is Project Release, located in New York City and started by a patient who was living in a neglected single-room occupancy hotel after he was released from a mental hospital. He organized a group of ex-patients to attempt to improve his situation and theirs. Together they found housing and, today, the original commune abandoned, Project Release operates out of a large apartment where its members serve as patient advocates for hundreds of former patients.

In its three and one-half years of operation, funded by donations and grants, Project Release has received calls and handled well over 1,000 cases. The group depends on lawyers of the New York Civil Liberties Union for help with legal problems. For example, if a patient wants release from a mental hospital and calls Project Release, a member, acting as a consumer advocate, calls the Civil Liberties Union for help in investigating the case and following through as the facts warrant.

By means of conferences held throughout the state and lectures by members, the goals of the Project, admittedly termed "radical" by members, are spelled out to ex-patients, their families, neighbors, and potential employers. The project strongly subscribes to the concept that treatment should be a matter of choice with mental patients or ex-patients, theirs to accept or reject as one of their rights. Project members point out that professional therapy may *not* be what a patient needs; the understanding of others may be of greater benefit.

Nursing Home Ombudsman

While self-help groups with a health focus are composed of special patient or ex-patient populations acting in their own interests, there are a number of programs that recognize the vulnerability of patients unable to organize or to advocate for their own needs. Especially vulnerable groups for whom special ombudsman and advocate services have been established are elderly, terminally ill, and handicapped individuals who are residents of nursing homes and other long-term care facilities.

Nursing home ombudsman programs are being reported in the literature with increasing frequency. Perhaps the greatest impetus came from Washington when, in 1973, the Department of Health, Education and Welfare (now Department of Health and Human Services), seeking to improve the care of nursing home residents and meet public clamor against their mistreatment, established a Nursing Home Ombudsman Demonstration Project. It was funded first in Wisconsin, Michigan, South Carolina, Pennsylvania, and Idaho and in 1974 was extended to Oregon and Massachusetts. Its purpose was "to invite and investigate complaints registered by patients and/or their families and friends regarding patient care."[10] As part of the project, a manual was produced which attempted to show how the ombudsman concept could be applied to a nursing home setting and illustrate some complaint-handling procedures and techniques. The nursing home ombudsmen in this project were described as independent, impartial, and necessarily expert in nursing home affairs. Like the classic ombudsman, these ombudsmen had the power to recommend changes and publicize abuses. Their principal charge was to help patients and families who questioned treatment received in a nursing home. Unlike the classical ombudsmen, they worked with no tradition in this country or legislated jurisdictional authority.

During the first year, the five demonstration projects set up by HEW received 1,196 complaints from 713 complainants, most of them made by friends or relatives acting for patients. Only a few complaints (7 percent) were about food. More than half concerned quality of care, administrative policies, and payment. About 80 percent of the complaints, in the judgment of ombudsmen and their consultants, were justified and could or should be corrected. It was estimated that complaints were resolved satisfactorily in 55 to 60 percent of the cases. The ombudsmen followed through with the appropriate regulatory or service agency to make sure that appropriate action was taken and remained in effect. This follow-up constituted a key factor in the success of the programs in the five projects. Among the problems identified as needing further action were: over-use of tranquilizers, inadequate physician care, inappropriate placement of patients, life-care contracts, excessive charges, and need for training of nursing home staff.[11]

In New York in 1975, acting in response to the reports of widespread abuses in nursing homes, the Moreland Commission on Nursing Homes recommended a patient advocate or ombudsman program, which was established by legislation administered by the New York State Health Commissioner. Ombudsmen were required ". . . to receive complaints of poor patient care or other deficiencies [in nursing homes] and to oversee immediate follow up investigations and corrective action."[12] A patient advocate was established in every county of the State. Less populated counties were to employ part-time advocates. In January 1977, the New York City patient advocate program started a "Hot Line" which operates 24 hours a day, including weekends, to handle patient complaints. Notices in nursing homes inform patients that they may reverse charges to Albany after ordinary business hours when the service operates by recording calls. The service covers hospitals and health-related facilities as well as nursing homes.

A state code outlines the powers of the advocate program. By written notice a facility is informed of impending action. Every complaint made by telephone or in writing receives an answer by letter. Site visits are usually made in response to a complaint about poor food or poor care in a nursing home. Sometimes billing complaints can be handled with a site visit, but they are the exceptions. Fines may run as high as $1,000 a day. About 100 nursing home, 75 to 80 hospital and 25 financial cases are handled a month, ranging from complaints about care to complaints against both doctors and nurses. A review conducted by the American Jewish Congress and the Community Action and Resources for the Elderly of the first two years of activity was highly critical of this program. It concluded that while the Office of Patient Advocate was a good idea, it was being strangled in its own red tape. On four separate counts the review found the program inefficient and indifferent to public needs: 1. Investigations were delayed and incomplete. 2. Political considerations were a factor in handling complaints. (For example, if the governor or a high public official forwarded the complaint, it received special attention.) 3. There was an absence of contact with complainants and a tendency to refer complaints to nursing home administrators. 4. Complainants often were judged instead of their complaints; that is, when the investigator found the patient "confused" or "disoriented" he often ignored a specific complaint such as theft of a patient's property.

The report did not suggest that the patient advocates be discontinued in nursing homes but, rather, that the position be strengthened by means of sufficient resources (money and staff) so as to better protect the rights of nursing home residents. It recommended that the patient advocates be made independent of government agencies and "empowered to take quick action to resolve complaints . . .," meet with patients and their families to explain their rights, and help develop mechanisms for assisting patients in the assertion and practice of these rights. The advocates would investigate all complaints, even of "disoriented" patients, work for patients, and devise ways of preventing fear of retaliation against a complaint. Legislation was recommended along the lines of that already enacted in relation to child abuse, which legally obligates physicians, nurses, and other personnel to report all cases of suspected abuse or maltreatment of patients. Critical as it was, the report saw a strengthened patient advocate system as a basic protector of the rights of men and women living out their days in nursing homes.[13]

Another approach to the protection of the rights of residents of nursing homes and other long-term care facilities has been the formation of voluntary organizations whose membership acts for them as their consumer advocates. These organizations are not intended to supplant the government sponsored nursing home ombudsman programs, but to identify residents with complaints or problems and to stimulate nursing home operators and government monitoring agencies to satisfactorily resolve their problems. A second function has been to identify class action issues affecting a sizeable group of residents and to exert pressure toward resolution by means of appeals to state legislators and the press and through legal action.

Citizens for Better Care, established in 1969 in Detroit, is one such voluntary organization. Its major concern is with monitoring nursing homes, homes for the aged, and residential after-care facilities for patients released from mental hospitals. Most of its membership are either retired individuals or professionals concerned with working with the aged. Operators of nursing homes are excluded from the organization in the interests of independence and because they are viewed as adversaries. The organization undertakes individual and class advocacy action. It receives telephone or written complaints about nursing homes and monitors these complaints until they are satisfactorily resolved. It acts as adversaries of the nursing home industry at legislative hearings, has initiated class action lawsuits and has stimulated coverage by the press of issues of importance in protecting the rights of nursing home residents. While originally financed by contributions from local churches, and operating in rent free quarters, it later expanded as funding was received from the Urban Coalition, the United States Department of Health, Education and Welfare, the Regional Medical Program, and other sources. The organization considers that it has made effective contributions by individual and class advocacy actions, by serving as a monitor of formal regulatory and inspection functions of government agencies, and by producing a series of studies used in planning and policy formation. It considers its success attributable to at least three factors: careful selection of issues to be pursued by its membership, use of the courts, and the financing of activities by funds supplied through government grants.[14]

An organization similar to Citizens for Better Care was established in New York City in 1976 as the Friends and Relatives of Institutionalized Aged (FRIA). Its organizational rationale was based on the conviction that activities to protect and improve the system of care for the aged in institutions required ongoing vigilance. It enlisted families of institutionalized aged as the most continuously interested citizen group in the monitoring of abuses and patterns of poor care, as well as in providing reports on the progress of institutions in making promised corrections. It has offered some measure of anonymity to individual complainants who might fear retaliation by focussing on institution-wide patterns of poor care. It also has engaged in class advocacy and reform activities as well as providing public information on nursing home matters.[15] Its unique quality is that it draws on the natural interests of families of those who are institutionalized to provide ongoing vigilance and offers them consumer strength through numbers and professional expertise.

Ombudsman Programs in Group Medical Practice

As the solo practice of medicine has declined, a number of forms of group medical practice have developed. These differ from each other in form and method of payment, but they have in common the curtailment or limitation of the traditional physician-patient relationship. Some of these group practice arrangements have developed ombudsman programs which may serve to supplement or augment former functions performed by the physicians.

Most group practices are private medical partnerships in which a group of physicians, all with the same specialty or with a series of different specialties, practice together, charging on a fee-for-service basis. They are, in effect, formal extentions of the popular pattern of office partnerships and offer to the physician economic advantages as well as control of hours of work and other benefits. To the patient they offer broader and easier access to care and a measure of coordination of services. The function of the ombudsman in this kind of setting varies from group to group, but might include such activities as responding to patients who complain about the quality of care, who cannot or do not follow through on the use of services offered, who have difficulty finding an appropriate physician within the group to treat their complaints, and those who are at special risk because of age, status, or type of illness. While referred to as "ombudsman" services by the group practice organization, their responsibilities are more facilitative and preventative than the monitoring of care.

The patient counselor or ombudsman at the St. Louis Park Medical Center is an example of this kind of program. Headed by a former staff nurse, the program serves a triage function for the group. The ombudsman evaluates a patient's need for an appointment, recognizing potentially serious medical problems which may demand immediate care. In less serious cases, the ombudsman may explain the need to wait for an appointment, or may refer the patient outside of the medical group center. Questions about insurance and fees are answered. In handling patient complaints, the counselor ombudsman informs the physician and administration both verbally and in writing and makes an attempt to resolve the problem for the patient. In the opinion of the group, the service provided by the counselor ombudsman improves patient relations, facilitates the accurate communication of patients' problem to physicians and the administrator, increases telephone efficiency by screening inquiries and random calls, and helps patients to move through the medical care system by channeling them to appropriate physicians and to other services.

Another form of group practice is the health maintenance organization (HMO) which renders comprehensive health services to a voluntarily enrolled consumer population on a prepaid, fixed capitation basis. Services are provided by physicians and other health professionals who are employees or are partners in the organized group. To physicians, the advantages are similar to other forms of group practice in terms of predictability of income and control of time. To patients the main advantage is guaranteed access to all medical services at a fixed cost no matter how extensive the need. It is to the economic advantage of the providers to keep patients healthy in order to minimize the use of service, and this presumably accrues to the benefit of patients.

Patient representatives are employed by some HMOs. In some states, notably Minnesota, HMOs are required by law to provide a complaint system for patients. Other functions of the program include triage, the collection and feedback of data about regularly recurring patient complaints to the group's management, and improving patient-staff relationships.

In the Minneapolis-St. Paul area, at the nonprofit Nicollet/Eitel Family plan, an HMO, a patient representative is the complainant's first contact. The patient representative also resolves some complaints while referring others: medical complaints go to the chief of service who forwards unresolved matters to an executive appeals board. Nonmedical complaints related to personnel, system, and plant, which are not settled by the patient representative or department head, go to a five-person review committee or an executive review board. This group meets formally on a quarterly basis and suggests policy changes to correct situations producing repeated complaints.

At each stage of the complaint system, the patient representative informs the complainant in writing of the progress or action taken and keeps written records for investigative bodies. Easy access is emphasized. Patients may telephone complaints any time of the day or night. One added feature consists of an internal auditing committee of patient representative and chief administrator to obtain information regarding the effectiveness of the complaint system. Opinions are solicited from complainants and by a random sampling of plan enrollees.

Another HMO with an ombudsman program is the Community

Health Program of Queens-Nassau Inc. A patient services coordinator functions actively, assisted by two patient service representatives, a full-time secretary, and added clerical help. Many of the 300 or so cases handled every month by patient representatives revolve around financial matters and complicated Blue Cross contracts which need interpretation. However, problems involving medical care are also handled. The coordinator establishes communication between patients and staff, going directly to the appropriate staff member with a problem, and in the case of repeated complaints about a physician, may talk to the medical director. Patients are encouraged to use the patient representative service by means of a welcome kit for new subscribers, a quarterly newsletter, and an open house for enrollees.

The Health Insurance Plan of Greater New York is a well-established New York State HMO which provides group medical care to municipal employees and other subscribers. In 1974 it announced the appointment of an ombudsman charged with the task of increasing subscriber satisfaction with the plan. Subscriber good will, humanitarian concerns, and equity were the designated purposes of the program. The ombudsman is unsalaried, independent of HIP's 26 local medical groups, and is assisted by a salaried staff. A patient's complaint must be made first to the local group and, if unresolved, may then be brought to the ombudsman who has the power to order the medical group to accept the ombudsman's decision. The ombudsman handles an average of 300 cases per year, about 60 percent of them related to service and 40 percent to financial reimbursement. Patients learn about the service through a subscriber bulletin mailed directly to them.

Blue Cross Ombudsman

Blue Cross programs were originally organized and controlled by the American Hospital Association, but are currently independent and beginning to exercise monitoring functions over their former benefactors, the hospitals. By virtue of its capacity to withhold reimbursement of bills incurred by its subscribers, it can exert some influence. A number of Blue Cross Plans have adopted the ombudsman concept, among them the Northeastern New York Plan. The program was established to meet the needs of subscribers who often do not make their complaints known while in the hospital for fear of retaliation. They frequently turn to Blue Cross, as provider of their hospital benefits, to register complaints. To handle these complaints, the ombudsman sets up lines of communication with hospital patient representatives or other hospital authorities. The ombudsman also meets with hospital patient representatives as a group to exchange ideas and information and to help to identify common problem areas. The Blue Cross ombudsman also contacts consumer groups, exploring how they perceive their health benefits and what preferences they have for further coverage.

Overview of the Ombudsman's Role in Settings Outside the Hospital

Depending on origin, sponsorship, and task, community-based ombudsman programs can vary from those hired by government to those employed to watch nursing homes; from insurance plan staff members to those working in HMOs; from nonpaid parents and families of patients to patients advocating for themselves. What have they in common?

Each must have a modicum of independence in order to evaluate service and help to identify injustices.

Each must devise a method of easy access for complainants to reach the ombudsman.

Each must investigate all complaints, those that are valid and those that may be unfounded. In this way the agency, administrator, professional, or employee is protected against unjustified charges and the complainant against unsatisfactory treatment.

Each must function without resorting to professionals or officials against whom complaints have been lodged.

Each investigates and reports but does not prosecute. The greatest power resides in public opinion.

Based on repeated complaints, each may utilize feedback of information and suggest policy changes and program improvement.

Some may suggest, sponsor, and initiate new services.

None solve nor claim to solve all problems. By and large, each is ancillary to other monitoring, inspecting and auditing procedures.[16]

References

1. Eugene Feingold. "Who Controls the Medical Care System." *Health Services, the Local Perspective.* Proceedings of the Academy of Political Science, 32:3, edited by Arthur Levin, New York, The Academy of Political Science, 1977.

2. Vincent Navarro. *Medicine Under Capitalism.* New York, Prodist, 1976.

3. Walter Gelhorn. *Ombudsman and Others: Citizen's Protectors in Nine Countries.* Cambridge, Harvard University Press, 1966.

4. Elihu Katz and Brenda Danet (Eds.). *Bureaucracy and the Public: A Reader in Official Relations.* New York, Basic Books, 1973, p. 399.

5. Walter Gelhorn. "Confining Public Administration Without Crippling It." In *Bureaucracy and the Public: A Reader in Official Relations.* Edited by Elihu Katz and Brenda Danet. New York, Basic Books, 1973; D.C. Rowat, *The Ombudsman: Citizen's Defender.* London, Allen and Unwin, 1965.

6. Margaret Stacey. "Consumer Complaint Procedures in the British National Health Service." *Social Science and Medicine* 8:8:429–439, 1974.

7. Alonzo S. Yerby. *British National Health Services Complaints Procedures.* Washington, D.C., U.S. Department of Health, Education and Welfare, Health Services Administration, Public Health Service, NIH-76.

8. Charles Grosser. *New Directions in Community Organizing: From Enabling to Advocacy.* New York, Praeger Publishers, 1973.

9. George Brager and Steven Holloway. *Changing Human Service Organizations.* New York, Free Press, 1978.

10. Patrick Linnane. *Ombudsman for Nursing Homes: Structure and Process.* Washington, D.C. U.S. Department of Health, Education and Welfare, Office of Human Development, Administration on Aging, 1974, p. 2.

11. Allan Forman. "The Nursing Home Ombudsman Demonstration Program." *Health Services Report* 89:2:129–133, March-April, 1974.

12. New York State Health Department. News Release, January 20, 1975.

13. *Patients and Their Complaints: a Critical Study of New York State's Nursing Home Ombudsman.* A Joint Report by the American Jewish Congress and Community Action and Resources for the Elderly, April, 1977.

14. Solomon G. Jacobson. "Assessment of Consumer Advocacy in Improving Nursing Home Care." Unpublished paper presented at the 29th Annual Scientific Meeting of the Gerontological Society, New York, October 14, 1976.

15. *Who Cares.* Friends and Relatives of the Institutionalized Aged, Inc. (undated brochure).

16. James E. Payne. "Ombudsman Roles for Social Workers." *Social Work* 17:-1:94–100, January, 1972.

Part III

Hospital Ombudsman:
An Innovative Advocacy Program

Chapter V

An Ombudsman in a Hospital: The Patient Representative

HELEN REHR AND RUTH RAVICH

Two models of service to troubled citizens have been the underpinnings of patient representative programs in hospitals. These are the Citizens' Advice Bureaus developed by the English in London during World War II to aid dislodged or distressed city residents, and the Scandinavian Ombudsman who deals with "citizens' grievances against bureaucracy" and "resolving citizens' unique individual problems with a depersonalized administration."[1, 2] Patient representative programs have combined some of the objectives from each of these concepts and, over time, some of the programs in hospitals in this country have added a range of special functions indigenous to the institution.

The rationale for such programs in large hospitals centered on the complexity of the institution and its locked-in boundaries of specialized services resulting in great fragmentation of care and specialization of services. A large number of different occupational groups from the most professional to unskilled workers function in hospital settings.[3] The increase in division of labor means more departments and very frequently more departmentalized thinking. All these factors lead to patients and their family members having to become involved with many people when they are least able to cope with them.[4] The complex structure taxes not only the people to be served, but also those who serve in it, in terms of being knowledgeable of the many services and their interconnective necessity. In addition to fractionated and fragmented services, which have developed indepth rather than inbreadth perception, the daily working organization of the institution is rife with other problems:

-an explosion and growing accumulation of information, which prevents any one staff member from knowing all current information, and the maintenance of specialized knowledge in varied repositories known only to specialists;

-a set of revolving doorways which tend to return an individual back into the street if he cannot identify his problem in institutional terms and language;

-institutional pathways, each requiring its own registration in bureaucratic terms of identifying information and documents relevant to insurance coverage, Medicaid, Medicare, Blue Shield, or Blue Cross;

-medical attention requiring an available medical chart, which has to be retrieved from distant medical record rooms;

-needed laboratory tests and x-ray services requiring patients to traverse a veritable labyrinth;

-multiple illnesses that are separately dealt with, each in its own specialty clinic;

-coordination of medical opinions, laboratory, x-ray, and other critical information that must be not only centralized to a chart, but also interpreted by experts to give the data their proper significance.

The development of a patient representative or ombudsman program is predicated on the failure of individuals in need and the power system or subsystem to make a satisfactory encounter. The problem may be lodged in the individual or the provider, or in both. Patient representative programs are a relatively new organizational mechanism developed to facilitate the delivery of services to individuals encountering obstacles within medical centers. They can enhance an institution's capacity to provide patients with highly technical, specialized, and skilled care. Patient representatives may function under many different titles: patient advocate, patient service coordinator, or ombudsman. Their responsibilities are directed toward making "available to patients, staff, and community organizations a centralized source of information about the hospital and its services and offer direct consultation, referral and advocacy."[5] Some patient representatives have organized into the Society of Patient Representatives of the American Hospital Association (Appendix I), which describes its purposes:

The patient representative's primary assignment is to serve as the liaison between patients and the institution as a whole and between the institution and the community it serves. . . . provide(s) a specific channel through which patients can seek solutions to problems, concerns and unmet needs.

As the patient's advocate . . . enable patients and families to obtain solutions to problems by acting in their behalf with administration or any department or service, coordinating among departments if necessary and recommending alternative policies and procedures in order to improve service to patients. As the institution's direct representative, . . . interpret(s) its philosophy, policies, procedures and services to patients, their families and visitors.[6]

Early forms of patient representative programs were found most frequently in acute care hospitals. They were lodged in such different organizational segments as administration, social work services, public relations, and volunteer programs, and were essentially oriented to offering hospitality and courtesy services or dealing with certain types of grievances and complaints. The growth of patient representative programs in their present form began in the latter part of the 1960s when there was increasing recognition by administrators of the possible benefits and advantages in centralizing patient-expressed problems and their resolutions in one program. In addition, a flurry of programs surfaced in the late 1960s and early 1970s in response to consumers' organized efforts to deal with the growing depersonalization of hospital and medical services. Many of the concerns were expressed in newspapers, national magazines, professional journals, and in televised reports. Some of the organizational efforts to deal with consumer concerns appeared in articles and stories bearing subtitles such as: "Fighting the Hospital System," "Patient Relations Program for Clinics," "Who Is There to Care?" "City Hospital Worries About Patient," "The Patients' Friend, A Link Between Humanity and Science," "Hospitals Strive to Improve Their Images," "The Hospital Ombudsman."

Published stories of programs spurred the expansion of patient representative programs in the 1970s. Some of the programs described in the articles were short-lived, unable to withstand the fiscal crises in health care which the country and its medical institutions faced in the early part of the 1970s. The first program to publish a report of its activities in a professional journal was established in January 1967 at the Mount Sinai Medical Center in New York City. This program, initiated under the aegis of the hospital's Department of Social Work Services, responded to the needs of an outpatient clinic population which had a large proportion of families living at or below the level of poverty, who suffered from poor housing and underemployment and often had the additional barrier to service of being non-English-speaking.

The Mount Sinai program's purposes were to provide access to hospital services for individuals who were having difficulty in obtaining them, develop a feedback system to the institution about obstacles to the delivery of service, and act as a liaison between hospital, patients, and community agencies.[7] The program has continued and has expanded its functions to cover hospitalized patients as well as the ambulatory.

Later in the same year, a similar program was begun at the Presbyterian-University Hospital in Pittsburgh. Its purpose was to promote a "mutually responsive relationship" between the hospital and the three neighborhoods served by it. It aimed at initiating action that would lower the barriers to health care services for the poor and encourage greater use of hospital facilities.[8]

A third program oriented toward the needs of the disadvantaged and minority populations was developed at Michael Reese Hospital in Chicago. Established as an emergency room program in 1969 at a time when inner city tensions were high, the program reflected the concern of both the institution and the community with problems and dissatisfactions of 60,000 patients the hospital treated yearly in its around-the-clock emergency room. The intent of the program was to provide nonmedical aid to patients as they waited for care, explain emergency room procedures, help patients to understand the reasons for delays when they occurred, and provide waiting relatives with information when patients were being treated. The ombudsman in this program, chosen by the community, served a bridging function between the hospital and the patient population.[9]

At the same time as these programs directed toward clinic patients were developing, other patient representative programs, which primarily served inpatient hospitalized populations, were being established. Some of these began as fund-raising efforts and offered special attention to private patients whose comfort and satisfaction might eventuate in financial support for the hospital. These were broadened during the early 1970s to include all patients and to focus on patient satisfaction and comfort with care rather than on fund-raising.

Other inpatient programs were initiated by hospital administrations to improve feedback and control of patient care problems. A patient representative program of this type developed at New York Hospital in New York City. An important aspect of this program was an attempt to solve system problems through the use of the patient representative who, as an assistant to the president of the hospital, had enough prestige and power to intervene with system problems.

Programs taking various forms began proliferating in hospitals in several parts of the country. While each program developed to meet the special needs of the individual hospital, they all had some features in common. All were patient oriented and responsive to patient complaints. They provided information about the hospital to patients and their families, and most channeled back to the hospital manager information about the needs expressed by the patients. Beyond these commonalities, they possessed many unique features and exercised a range of functions.

Information and Referral

Most patient representatives perform information and referral functions within the hospital, and some offer information about community resources. In making these services available they may be individual-oriented or staff-oriented. In some programs, the information function is broadened to include communication via brochures and flyers, posters, and, in some cases, by group meetings of patients. This latter method is used most often to orient small groups of patients or family members to some aspect of hospital or medical care. In conjunction with information-giving, referrals are a logical sequence in the service pattern. In a few programs, advocacy on behalf of patients is a function of the patient representative. However, within the setting, advocacy more frequently takes the form of active persuasion. These functions are illustrated with the following:

1. Information

Patients who are in the halls or clinic waiting areas may ask the representatives for help or for information. Random visits to noncomplaining patients also elicit needs. A patient may feel ashamed or afraid to make a formal request or complaint, but when a representative comes to him, he is apt to talk about his concerns. For instance, a patient who at first hello says, "Everything is just fine" will very often say: "But I did notice," or "I would like. . . ." as a conversation continues. Other concerns are expressed in relation to any complexity or problem the individual has encountered within the institution, such as "how to become a registered patient," "unclear about a bill," or "the patient's status in regard to Medicare or Medicaid."

Requests for information and assistance by patients and families are also received by means of a "Hot Line" available in some hospitals on inpatient telephones. Patient orientation to nursing units may include an explanation of the patient representative program. If other programs are available, a paragraph in the patient information packets describes the functions and availability of the representative and the "Hot Line." In the outpatient department, visibility is achieved by a patient representative office with a large sign in an area through which ambulatory patients pass. In addition, other information is offered in relation to individualized need in the form of brochures and pamphlets; for example, on baby care, or in regard to services in the community, such as the local department of welfare.

2. Referral and Steering

Patients are seen by representatives on the basis of self-referral and by referral from medical, nursing, ancillary and administrative staff, and from such community organizations as churches, schools, social agencies, police and legal sources, and even television action reporters.

The availability and visibility of a patient representative on patient units and in the clinics on a regular basis provides another important referral source. When a patient representative is seeing a patient or making rounds, staff members often suggest a visit with other patients. The need for assistance may not seem sufficient for staff members to call a representative, but when available they are asked to help. Patients referred in this manner are often found to have serious concerns. As nursing staff members become aware of the representative's ability to open communications between departments, they seek help not only for patients but also with such off-unit problems, as getting reports and checking on test schedules.

Referrals may also be made to outside community social services on the basis of need. Information-giving and referral involve steering as well as motivating an individual to make contact and use the resource suggested. Follow-up as to whether the referral was used and was effective may be a part of the service.

An aspect of the information and referral function involves interdepartmental coordination. In highly complex hospitals in which the need for coordination and collaboration between departments is crucial, mechanisms may be set up to provide for integration.[10] Some patient representative functions include this form of integration. With patient complaints and problems as a data base, interdepartmental obstacles to providing effective service can be uncovered and brought to the attention of appropriate hospital authorities. In one hospital a problem that came to the attention of the patient representative resulted from the fact that two patients who were admitted on the same day had the same first and last names. The difficulties that are likely to occur are obvious. In an effort to determine if this was a common occurrence, the patient representative was able to secure a survey by the communications department of the administrative sector. During a one-month study, it appeared that 10 patients (five pairs) could be expected to have the same first and last names. In order to safeguard reports, medications, tests, and treatments, the departments of admitting, nursing, and communication developed a system of armband identification for patients with the same names. The capability of changing policies and procedures and improving structure lies with the medical and administrative decision makers, but a patient representative can act as a catalyst and/or facilitator.[11] A representative can be effective in bringing a patient's perceptions of care to the attention of staff members at all levels.

In other aspects of the information and referral function, a patient representative acts as a spokesperson for the hospital. This may take the form of public relations in terms of providing information that communicates the viewpoint of the hospital. Often, hospital rules and regulations as well as a patient's rights and privileges are provided in written form to entering patients, and the patient representative is designated as the individual to contact with requests or complaints. Hospital policy is explained to patients as important in achieving the goals for efficient and effective care, as well as in the patient's best interest.

Patient's Bill of Rights

Informing patients of their rights is new to the hospital field. Confronted with the problems and discontents expressed by patients, many institutions have introduced formal statements governing patients' rights. The American Hospital Association holds such statements as a standard expectation that must be readily available to patients and/or their family members as they are prepared to accept services from the institution:

> "In 1973, the AHA pioneered in the area of patients' rights . . . setting forth guidelines for hospitals . . . (for) ethical and procedural features of high quality of health care."[12]

The Bill of Rights has now been endorsed by many state legislatures in the country. In such instances, promulgation by the hospital is mandated. While "rights" have been stated in different ways by different medical institutions and the American Hospital Association, they cover common ground. (See Figure I for the most current statement issued by the Joint Commission on Accreditation of Hospitals.)

Patient representatives in a number of institutions orient staff members to the meaning of these rights and their implications for staff-patient interaction. In many staff meetings the *Patient's Bill of Rights* serves as a take-off point for sensitizing staff members to patient needs, feelings, and perceptions.

Hospitality and Courtesy Services

In some inpatient hospitality programs, patient representatives are like receptionists, visiting or greeting patients as they are admitted to the hospital and trying to make them comfortable while they await the real purpose of the visit. Representatives try to humanize the hospital experience by helping people understand what is happening to them and why rules and procedures are necessary. The warmth of a personal contact and an explanation help to put patients at ease and encourage compliance with hospital routines.

Two variants of this role occur frequently. One is the patient visitor role. In this role, representatives usually serve the inpatient population of the hospital and makes sure that patients are getting the housekeeping or "contact" services they are entitled to: hot food, clean sheets, and reasonably prompt attention to requests. The sister-visitors in Catholic hospitals, who often fulfill this role, also supply support and religious counseling to patients and families. Patient representatives are frequently asked to do errands for bed-bound patients. These may include having legal papers Xeroxed, securing a notary public, and even getting books or library services or therapeutic and recreational activities to patients.

In a second variant of this role, patient representatives serve as liaison between the operating room and families, providing information which can be reassuring, and locating physicians for family members.

Grievances, Complaints and Advocacy

Many programs have an additional major function: responding to grievances about the medical care and attitudes of hospital staff. These patient representative roles are modeled after the ombudsman or advocate role. Ombudsmen traditionally are accountable to an authority outside of the structure and are objective and impartial mediators. A patient representative, like an ombudsman, tries to be highly visible and accessible to patients, accepting and investigating complaints that arise from patients' encounters with any part of the hospital system. Patient representatives are expected to have access to any service staff person. As a result of a review of the facts, they can make recommendations to all categories of hospital personnel. While they have no power to enforce or coerce, the prestige of the position in an institution can be used to solve problems for patients and make recommendations for change.

In contrast to an ombudsman who makes impartial judgments about the claims from either the citizen or the organization, advocates unequivocally act to guard and promote the rights and interests of their clients but, at the same time, make an effort to maintain a nonadversary relationship with hospital staff. The idea of advocacy gained considerable attention in the 1960s. The advocate was seen as an individual with specific skills and expertise who could actively intercede and support disadvantaged individuals in order to help them gain access to services from which they might be barred. While patient representatives are sometimes called advocates and do act as such in behalf of relatively powerless patients, seldom are they expected to take the side of patients under all circumstances. A much more common pattern is for a patient representative to evaluate a patient's complaint and while pursuing those considered reasonable, also deal with the patient's perception of the causes. While a true advocate allows a client to maintain the prerogative for decision-making about what is to be pursued, a patient representative usually is more active in the problem-solving process.

Advocating in behalf of patients and their need for service is more frequently done in the context of persuasion or negotiation within a medical center than with confrontation or demand. Patient representatives, because they are located within the establishment, need to keep present and future channels of communication open to them. Therefore, the role in safeguarding a patient's service is done by achieving the linkage through facilitative means, including securing reports, opening communication with staff members, and speaking in a patient's behalf.

Both in the ombudsman and advocacy roles, there are limits on the methods and goals at the disposal of patient representatives because of their position as employees within the hospital structure. In effect, hospitals have institutionalized the role of advocate or ombudsman in the form of patient representation. This has placed limitations on the scope and the methods at its disposal. Patient representatives' major techniques are communication, data gathering, education, persuasion, and negotiation. Coercive or adversary modes of intervention are beyond their scope. A patient representative can be effective as long as what the patient wants or needs and what the hospital is willing or able to provide are fairly consonant. Redress of grievances and even changes in procedures and policies are usually possible under these conditions.

The advantage of hospital-based patient representatives is that with knowledge of the system, they have the capacity to use formal as well as informal channels to achieve appropriate services or benefits for patients. They also are available to deal with and solve problems as they occur. However, if what a patient demands exceeds what the hospital is capable or willing to provide, the conflict is beyond the scope of a patient representative. Adjudicating techniques must then come into play, and patients then are better served through the legal system or by an advocate not accountable to and paid for by the hospital. Adjudications can be offered following review of complaints by a professional society, such as the geographically-relevant medical society, or by state professional examination boards or the more recently instituted state ombudsman or quality assurance committee. In some instances other adversary measures are instituted by patients who seek redress through the courts.

The Risk Management Function

An emerging role of patient representatives is in risk management. In this role, found mostly in grievance-type patient representative programs, the patient representative intervenes, usually as one member of a committee, in responding to situations which may lead to malpractice suits. This includes investigating incidents, reviewing reports, talking to patients, families, and staff and making appropriate recommendations. There are three categories of incidents with which a patient representative as a member of the risk management team may deal. The first category is one where the primary complaint centers around incidents in which a patient claims irreversible damage was incurred during the hospital stay. A patient representative may be assigned to make initial investigations of these incidents, establishing factual data, assessing the complainant's attitude toward the institution, and making recommendations for action. A second category of incidents is that in which minor or reversible damage to a patient has been claimed, particularly complaints about medical mismanagement that do not lead to permanent damage or discomfort, discourtesies, and inconvenience as well as loss of property. Patient representatives attempt to resolve some of these problems and/or allay the patient's anger. An assumption is made that when a damaging event has occurred, a patient who is angry at the hospital or its staff may react with greater propensity to sue. A supposition, requiring research, is that a patient representative may be able to reduce the number of malpractice actions by responding in an individualized way to the aggrieved patient, such as making adjustments in billing, arranging for replacement of lost items, and alerting staff members that extra attention and consideration must be rendered.

A third category of incidents is one that on the surface appear not likely to eventuate in a malpractice action by a patient, but which reveal a pattern of patient care that has the potential for creating problems in the future. A patient representative may continually investigate and document these and channel information back to appropriate departments or to administration.

Community Liaison Services

Another variant more often found in outpatient programs than in inpatient programs is the indigenous community representative who acts as a bridge, linking the hospital to community residents who use its facilities. Some of these programs, directed primarily at poverty level and minority groups, attempt to remove the barriers to service occasioned by the gap between the hospital professionals and the patients. In some programs the purpose also is to reduce tension between neighborhood groups and the hospital. Indigenous community leaders who might potentially be instrumental in community protest were sometimes hired or sought as community board volunteers in order to coopt them and reduce community conflict but, more currently, to seek out the opinions of those with similar backgrounds as that of the patients served.[13]

A patient representative based in the hospital may be called upon to respond to community requests. Inquiries about the hospital's facilities and programs may result in providing tours of the institution for community groups. Talks on specialized subjects and services may be given to neighborhood groups. Arranging for preschool, precamp, and preemployment physical examinations can be a hospital's means of relating more closely with community agencies that make such requests. Agency staff members feel very positively about having a centralized information resource within the hospital to respond to the health care requests of their clientele.

The Accounts Representative

Still another role is carried by individuals who use the title of patient representative, although these representatives bear little in common with those who are members of the Society of Patient Representatives. Essentially, these patient representatives function as financial officers. The hospital assigns each patient to a representative who then is responsible for all financial activities in relation to admissions, discharges, insurance, and credit.[14] The goal is to improve the collection of funds by reducing the numbers of people to whom a patient must relate in working out financial problems. The Society of Patient Representatives—the national membership organization of patient representatives, a subsidiary of the American Hospital Association—is currently attempting to clarify the title of "patient representative" to clearly exclude this financial function.

Patient representative programs, thus, have taken on a range of functions and roles in general hospitals. A few hospitals include all the activities noted. In the majority, one or more function may be in the patient representative job description. In whatever form, these programs are becoming increasingly common in short-term hospitals, especially those with over 200 beds and teaching hospitals. They have been mandated in some government institutions.

In addition to the functions already discussed, the tools of patient representatives should include skills essential for high quality performance. They must be good listeners with an ability to be empathic, yet open enough so as not to take sides. It is critical for representatives to be thoroughly knowledgeable about the workings of the institution, its varied personnel, and the nature of their interrelationships. A representative needs to be able to move fully within all echelons of the medical center. The representative has two major functions: ". . . to 'troubleshoot' for the patient who has become entangled in the red tape of complex hospital procedures, and to develop a system of feedback to appropriate staff members regarding some of the innumerable obstacles that have developed within the institution to delay or prevent the delivery of comprehensive . . . services to patients."[15]

Feedback

In order to modify programs that may be creating unanticipated obstacles to the delivery of services, a patient representative must collect data. A central place for complaints and problems provides data about patients' perceptions of care. A profile of patient experiences needs to be compiled from the information received from patients, their families, staff, community and governmental agencies, hospital incident reports, complaints and commendation letters received by the administration, and comments written on patient post-discharge questionnaires. Periodic analysis of these data provides information about the climate in patient-care areas of the hospital. Documentation with a data base permits a representative to meet with appropriate department personnel "with specific information relating to . . . impediments to giving service to patients."[16] Information that is gathered by patient representatives concerning problems experienced by patients contributes to overall evaluation of programs and thus serves as a ready administrative tool.

Assessment and Recommendations

An examination of patient representative programs in medical centers shows that their major achievements are in behalf of individuals who have encountered problems in care. Programs have demonstrated a capability of working on a one-to-one basis with staff members so as to modify former resistance or open the door to a service. In addition, staff at the service level and community agencies' representatives tend to be gratified with the facilitating services provided by patient representation. The results are more mixed with regard to securing service changes. Some staff members in authority are extremely responsive to learning about delivery problems, and may even draw on a patient representative for suggestions regarding training or procedural changes. In some cases any implication of impediments in service delivery has been resisted, with a range of responses from indifference, hostility, to "it's not timely" or the personnel is "not up to change." There are critics who indicate that a patient representative does no more than "cool" the issues by helping to resolve individual problems, and they believe that patient representatives may in essence be a reason for prolonging the change process. Some administrators believe situations should be allowed to "deteriorate" or "break-down", so as to avoid bypassing, temporizing, or ameliorating the conflict. Critics also question whether there can be true impartiality as long as a patient representative is based within the hospital. This is sometimes answered by suggesting that both hospitals and patients have the same goal, that is, good patient care, and that a patient representative can successfully maintain the dual orientation required by impartiality. This assumption is open to question. However, it is important to keep in mind that a patient representative is capable of responding objectively to a large number of patient situations, especially those in which a conflict of "territorial" interests is not a prominent element.

When quality communication is achieved between patient and provider, many problems disappear. However, some form of programs, such as informed counseling, advocacy, referral, and even health education in the medical setting will be more in demand in the future as patient representative programs continue to demonstrate their value to both patients and the institution. A complex institution has an obligation to provide internal mechanisms for dealing with breakdown in services so that sound access to health care is the right of every patient.

Rights and Responsibilities of Patients *

The basic rights of human beings for independence of expression, decision, and action, and concern for personal dignity and human relationships are always of great importance. During sickness, however, their presence or absence become vital, deciding factors in survival and recovery. Thus it becomes a prime responsibility for hospitals to assure that these rights are preserved for their patients.

In providing care, hospitals have the right to expect behavior on the part of patients, their relatives and friends, which, considering the nature of their illness, is reasonable and responsible.

This statement does not presume to be all-inclusive. It is intended to convey the Joint Commission's concern about the relationship between hospitals and patients, and to emphasize the need for the observance of the rights and responsibilities of patients.

The following basic rights and responsibilities of patients are considered reasonably applicable to all hospitals.

Patient Rights

ACCESS TO CARE

Individuals shall be accorded impartial access to treatment or accommodations that are available or medically indicated, regardless of race, creed, sex, national origin, religion, or sources of payment for care.

RESPECT AND DIGNITY

The patient has the right to considerate, respectful care at all times and under all circumstances, with recognition of his personal dignity.

PRIVACY AND CONFIDENTIALITY

The patient has the right, within the law, to personal and informational privacy, as manifested by the right to:

- refuse to talk with or see anyone not officially connected with the hospital, including visitors, or persons officially connected with the hospital but who are not directly involved in his care.

- wear appropriate personal clothing and religious or other symbolic items, as long as they do not interfere with diagnostic procedures or treatment.
- be interviewed and examined in surroundings designed to assure reasonable audiovisual privacy. This includes the right to have a person of one's own sex present during certain parts of a physical examination, treatment, or procedure performed by a health professional of the opposite sex; and the right not to remain disrobed any longer than is required for accomplishing the medical purpose for which the patient was asked to disrobe.
- expect that any discussion or consultation involving his case will be conducted discreetly, and that individuals not directly involved in his care will not be present without his permission.
- have his medical record read only by individuals directly involved in his treatment or the monitoring of its quality, and by other individuals only on his written authorization or that of his legally authorized representative.
- expect all communications and other records pertaining to his care, including the source of payment for treatment, to be treated as confidential.
- request a transfer to another room if another patient or visitors in that room are unreasonably disturbing him by smoking or other actions.
- be placed in protective privacy when considered necessary for personal safety.

PERSONAL SAFETY

The patient has the right to expect reasonable safety insofar as the hospital practices and environment are concerned.

IDENTITY

The patient has the right to know the identity and professional status of individuals providing service to him, and to know which physician or other practitioner is primarily responsible for his care. This includes the patient's right to know of the existence of any professional relationship among individuals who are treating him, as well as the relationship to any other health care or educational institutions involved in his care. Participation by patients in clinical training programs or in the gathering of data for research purposes should be voluntary.

INFORMATION

The patient has the right to obtain from the practitioner responsible for coordinating his care, complete and current information concerning his diagnosis (to the degree known), treatment, and any known prognosis. This information should be communicated in terms the patient can reasonably be expected to understand. When it is not medically advisable to give such information to the patient, the information should be made available to a legally authorized individual.

COMMUNICATION

The patient has the right of access to people outside the hospital by means of visitors, and by verbal and written communication.

When the patient does not speak or understand the predominant language of the community, he should have access to an interpreter. This is particularly true where language barriers are a continuing problem.

CONSENT

The patient has the right to reasonably informed participation in decisions involving his health care. To the degree possible, this should be based on a clear, concise explanation of his condition and of all proposed technical procedures, including the possibilities of any risk of mortality or serious side effects, problems related to recuperation, and probability of success. The patient should not be subjected to any procedure without his voluntary, competent, and understanding consent, or that of his legally authorized representative. Where medically significant alternatives for care or treatment exist, the patient shall be so informed.

The patient has the right to know who is responsible for authorizing and performing the procedures or treatment.

The patient shall be informed if the hospital proposes to engage in or perform human experimentation or other research/educational projects affecting his care or treatment, and the patient has the right to refuse to participate in any such activity.

CONSULTATION

The patient, at his own request and expense, has the right to consult with a specialist.

REFUSAL OF TREATMENT

The patient may refuse treatment to the extent permitted by law. When refusal of treatment by the patient or his legally authorized representative prevents the provision of appropriate care in accordance with ethical and professional standards, the relationship with the patient may be terminated upon reasonable notice.

TRANSFER AND CONTINUITY OF CARE

A patient may not be transferred to another facility unless he has received a complete explanation of the need for the transfer and the alternatives to such a transfer, and unless the transfer is acceptable to the other facility. The patient has the right to be informed by the responsible practitioner or his delegate of any continuing health care requirements following discharge from the hospital.

HOSPITAL CHARGES

Regardless of the source of payment for his care, the patient has the right to request and receive an itemized and detailed explanation of his total bill for services rendered in the hospital. The patient has the right to timely notice prior to termination of his eligibility for reimbursement by any third-party payer for the cost of his care.

HOSPITAL RULES AND REGULATIONS

The patient should be informed of the hospital rules and regulations applicable to his conduct as a patient. Patients are entitled to information about the hospital's mechanism for the initiation, review, and resolution of patient complaints.

Patient Responsibilities PROVISION OF INFORMATION

A patient has the responsibility to provide, to the best of his knowledge, accurate and complete information about present complaints, past illnesses, hospitalizations, medications, and other matters relating to his health. He has the responsibility to report unexpected changes in his condition to the responsible practitioner. A patient is responsible for making it known whether he clearly comprehends a contemplated course of action and what is expected of him.

COMPLIANCE WITH INSTRUCTIONS

A patient is responsible for following the treatment plan recommended by the practitioner primarily responsible for his care. This may include following the instructions of nurses and allied health personnel as they carry out the coordinated plan of care and implement the responsible practitioner's orders, and as they enforce the applicable hospital rules and regulations. The patient is responsible for keeping appointments and, when he is unable to do so for any reason, for notifying the responsible practitioner or the hospital.

REFUSAL OF TREATMENT

The patient is responsible for his actions if he refuses treatment or does not follow the practitioner's instructions.

HOSPITAL CHARGES

The patient is responsible for assuring that the financial obligations of his health care are fulfilled as promptly as possible.

HOSPITAL RULES AND REGULATIONS

The patient is responsible for following hospital rules and regulations affecting patient care and conduct.

RESPECT AND CONSIDERATION

The patient is responsible for being considerate of the rights of other patients and hospital personnel, and for assisting in the control of noise, smoking, and the number of visitors. The patient is responsible for being respectful of the property of other persons and of the hospital.

*Accreditation Manual for Hospitals, 1980 Edition, Joint Commission on Accreditation of Hospitals, Chicago, Illinois, pp. xiii-xvi.

References

1. Alfred J. Kahn et al. *Neighborhood Information Centers: A Study and Some Proposals.* New York, Columbia University Press, 1966, pp. 33–35.

2. H.S. Reuss and S.V. Anderson. "The Ombudsman: Tribune of the People." *Annals of the American Academy of Political Social Science* 363:1:44–51, Jan. 1966.

3. Herbert E. Klarman. *The Economics of Health.* New York, Columbia University Press, 1965, p. 4.

4. Richard M. Titmuss. *Essays on the Welfare State.* New Haven, Yale University Press, 1959, pp. 123–128.

5. R.W. Ravich, H. Rehr, and C.H. Goodrich. "Ombudsman: A New Concept in Voluntary Hospital Services." *Human Services and Social Work Responsibil-*

ity. Edited by Willard C. Richan. New York, National Association of Social Workers, 1969, p. 313.

6. The Society of Patient Representatives, "A Descriptive Definition." Chicago, mimeographed, undated, Chapter VI.

7. Ruth W. Ravich, Helen Rehr, and Charles H. Goodrich. "Hospital Ombudsman Smooths Flow of Service and Communications." *Hospitals* 43:5:56–61, March 1, 1969.

8. Eugene Vodev. "Reaching Out to the Poor." *Hospitals* 47:70–72, August 11, 1973.

9. Richard Cavalier. "Ombudsman is Middle Man Between Clinic Patients and Hospital." *Modern Hospital* 114:1:92, January 1970.

10. Paul Lawrence and Jay Lorsch. *Developing Organizations: Diagnosis and Action.* Reading, Mass., Addison-Wesley Publishing Company, 1969, p. 13.

11. Ruth Ravich and Helen Rehr. "Ombudsman Program Provides Feedback." *Hospitals* 48:18:63–67, September 16, 1974.

12. Patients' Rights, in American Hospital Association, Review of the Year 1973 (Chicago, Ill.), p. 20.

13. Paul A. Kurzman. "The New Careers Movement and Social Change." *Social Casework* 51:1:22–27, January 1970.

14. Studs Terkel. *Working.* New York, Avon Books, 1972, pp. 646–650.

15. R. Ravich, H. Rehr, and C.H. Goodrich. *Op. cit., Hospitals,* p. 43.

16. *Ibid.* p. 55.

Chapter VI

Models For Patient Representative Programs

Mildred D. Mailick

Background

The idea of a patient representative program has evoked much interest among hospitals all over the United States and abroad. The Society of Patient Representatives reports that it receives an average of fifty inquiries per month asking for information and help by hospitals wishing to initiate programs. Some directors of patient representative programs in large urban hospitals report that they also devote considerable time to interviews with representatives of hospitals that are starting programs of their own and are seeking to benefit from the experience of those already established.

A manual published by the Society of Patient Representatives of the American Hospital Association in 1978 provides guidelines for setting up patient representative programs, but there is relatively little current information upon which to base decisions about the type of program to develop.

The Society of Patient Representatives gathers personal and program data about its own members each year, but their data base does not include the large number of individuals and programs unaffiliated with the national organization. In fact, until 1975 there was little exact information about the number of programs actually functioning in hospitals. At that time a question was included in a special survey conducted by the American Hospital Association which reached almost all hospitals in the United States and asked each if it had a functioning patient representative program. While 1,447 of over 7,000 hospitals replied affirmatively, the definition of patient representative used in the survey was so nebulous that the replies were of little value. The American Hospital Association at that time defined a patient representative simply as a person "who serves as liaison between patients and hospital." This overly inclusive definition led many hospitals to reply that they had patient representative programs.

They were later found to have reported programs of other kinds that in some way *did* involve liaison with the patients, but were not concerned with a patient complaint function. Only about two-thirds of the hospitals reporting patient representative programs in this special survey fell within the more specific definition later developed by the Society of Patient Representatives:

> The patient representative's primary assignment is to serve as the liaison between patients and the institution as a whole and between the institution and the community it serves. They provide a specific channel through which patients can seek solutions to problems, concerns and unmet needs.
>
> As the patient's advocate they enable patients and families to obtain solutions to problems by acting in their behalf with administration or any department or service, coordinating among departments if necessary and recommending alternative policies and procedures in order to improve service to patients.
>
> As the institution's direct representative, they interpret its philosophy, policies, procedures and services to patients, their families and visitors.[1]

In addition to lack of knowledge about the number of patient representative programs, there were few specifics about the characteristics of programs in different sizes and types of hospitals, nor was there much information about the functions performed by programs of different types.

The President's Committee on Medical Malpractice Study

An early study conducted in 1971–1972 threw some light on these questions. The President's Committee on Medical Malpractice conducted a *Study of Patient Grievance Mechanisms* that contained data derived from a nationwide survey. The study attempted to locate and analyze a variety of patient grievance mechanisms found at all levels of administration in long-term and short-term hospitals and other health care organizations. A questionnaire was sent to 2,200 health care institutions in the United States. About one-half (1,050), mostly from states east of the Mississippi, responded; and 280 (27 percent) of these reported patient grievance mechanisms of one kind or another. Of this group of 280 institutions, 92 or one-third had job titles which were subsumed under the title of "patient complaint function," while the rest appeared to have titles of administrator (considered to be part of top management) or directors of public or patient relations. Because the analysis was based on job titles rather than on job functions or activities, it is difficult to determine exactly how well what is described as the "patient complaint function" coincides with the patient representative programs as defined by the Society of Patient Representatives. Nevertheless, the study did provide information about characteristics of hospitals and characteristics of grievance mechanism programs that existed at the time of the study, and also made recommendations about the establishment of further grievance programs in hospitals and other health care agencies.

Data from this study reveal that patient greivance programs were most likely to be found in voluntary hospitals of over 200 beds. The patient complaint function, that is, the program closest in characteristics to the patient representative, appeared, in general, to be at a lower level in the organizational hierarchy as compared to other programs described in the study. Those working in patient complaint programs tended to be more poorly paid (under $15,000 per year), had less education than others in the hierarchy, and were more likely to be women. The study included data derived from on-site visits to a small group of the hospitals.

A number of factors were found to influence the development of patient grievance programs. One was the loss of charitable immunity during the 1960s by many hospitals. Administrators of these hospitals were confronted with an increased possibility of legal suits, and sought to reduce their vulnerability by developing patient grievance programs. Some of the hospitals sought new mechanisms for increasing the ability of the patients to be heard. Postdischarge questionnaires, which gave the patients an opportunity to express their response to the care that was received in the hospital, were supplanted or supplemented by new patient grievance programs which sought to obtain complaints from patients while they were still in the hospital and while the complaints might be resolved satisfactorily. Some programs in large hospitals were initiated as "trouble shooting" mechanisms to respond to system dysfunction and to recommend changes in hospital procedures. The admissions process was a special source of trouble, and many of the programs were directed specifically to patients as they entered the hospital. Other programs were directed at special population groups. One group of hospitals provided special personalized services to "VIP" patients: celebrities or those who might possibly support the hospital financially. Lower income, minority patients were another special population served by programs, especially in outpatient departments and emergency rooms where the programs were directed at improving or maintaining good community relations. In sum, this study describes a range of programs that reflected the beginnings of patient representative mechanisms.

A number of other more modest studies were conducted which, while specifically directed toward patient representative programs, were hampered by being based on a smaller number of hospitals or were not based on a representative sample. For example, several questionnaire studies drew a sample of programs from the membership list of the Society of Patient Representatives. The data from these studies could not accurately reflect the range of programs in the United States because they were biased by the fact that those who affiliate with national organizations tend to be a self-selected group, and differ in important ways from their unaffiliated colleagues. Other studies were based on hospitals in a single geographical area, and represented regional biases. The remaining published accounts of patient representative programs that appeared in journals were descriptive in form, and tended to note how one program developed in a specific setting.

The Survey of Patient Representative Study

In 1975–1976 another study was conducted which tried to deal with some of these problems.[3] The study gathered baseline data about patient representative programs located in short-term general hospitals in the continental United States. Since it was not confined to members of the Society for Patient Representatives, it was more representative in scope than some of the previous studies. It was based on a sample of 448 hospitals, stratified by size and geographical area, that reported a patient representative program functioning during the calendar year of 1974.

The questionnaire was designed to explore specific characteristics of patient representative programs. It was directed to the person assuming major responsibility for conducting the patient representative program, and the hospital administrator was asked to determine who that person was. It was divided into four sections: 1. A series of questions about the characteristics of the patient representative program including how it was currently staffed and funded and how its activities were reported. 2. Personal data about the patient representative who assumed major responsibility for conducting the program, including age, sex, salary and education. 3. Information on referral and coverage patterns of the programs. 4. A list of 28 activities considered to be the principal tasks of the patient representatives. In addition to data about the patient representative program derived from the questionnaire, a profile of characteristics about each hospital in the study was drawn from the data files of the American Hospital Association. These included the size of hospital, its location in an urban or rural community, type of control (governmental, voluntary or for profit) and whether the hospital was a teaching or nonteaching hospital.

Of the sample of 448 hospitals in the study, 347 responded to the questionnaire, and 217 (62.5 percent) of the responding hospitals reported a currently functioning patient representative program. The results of the study suggested that patient representative programs were more likely to be in hospitals located in larger urban than in smaller rural areas, in teaching rather than non-teaching hospitals, and in voluntary as opposed to governmental or for profit institutions. These data support the idea that the larger, more complex hospitals were searching for mechanisms to humanize their services and to develop a more personalized link with patients. The study also reveals that most patient representative programs were relatively new to the hospital scene. Over 81 percent had been established since 1970, and the rate of increase accelerated with each year. By 1976, one in every five hospitals in the United States had a patient representative program, and in hospitals with over 500 beds, it was one of every two hospitals.

The financing of patient representative programs also proved to be interesting. Over 90 percent were funded through the regular hospital budget, rather than from outside grants. In addition, three-fourths of the programs reported to the central administrator's department. This suggests that most of the programs studied had limited independence as they were heavily dependent on hospital administrators.

The size and coverage of the programs were also investigated. Most were quite small. Almost three-fourths had staffs of two or less. Almost all of the larger programs were located in hospitals with 300 or more beds. Volunteers were used in 30 percent of the programs, and tended to be more common in urban hospitals. Over 96 percent of the programs offered services to inpatients, either alone or in combination with services to other areas of the hospital. Less than 4 percent offered services only in outpatient areas (emergency rooms and clinics).

Salary levels and educational preparation of the patient representative group at the time of the study suggest that they occupied relatively middle-level positions in the hospital hierarchy. Forty-three percent earned under $10,000, over one-third had no more than a high school education, 80 percent were women, over 50 percent had been working as patient representatives for less than four years, and almost 66 percent were already employed in their hospitals prior to the creation of the programs.

Perhaps the most important finding of this study was the identification of the types of activities patient representatives performed (See Table 1). Almost 90 percent of the patient representative programs reported that three activities were performed very often or fairly often: providing information about hospital services to patients and family groups, investigating and/or directing inquiries and complaints to appropriate hospital staff, and collecting data and channeling information about recurring patient care problems to appropriate hospital services. These can be considered the core activities of patient representative programs.

Four activities are reported as occurring seldom or not at all by at least 60 percent of the hospitals: participating in community meetings and on community boards, acting as advocate in complaints to the hospital administration on behalf of community groups, independently adjusting bills within specified limits, and acting as assigned representative for patients' accounts. These activities can be considered peripheral to most

Table 1

Frequency of Activities Performed By Patient Representative Programs

Activity	Very Often %	Fairly Often %	Seldom or Never %	Total %
Hospitality	44.3	22.2	33.5	100.0
Information to patients/families	74.4	21.4	4.2	100.0
Information to community groups	19.9	30.4	49.7	100.0
Investigates complaints	65.9	29.4	4.7	100.0
Community meetings	11.7	25.2	63.1	100.0
Translation	14.4	31.1	54.5	100.0
Transportation	18.4	27.2	54.4	100.0
Other services	44.2	39.9	15.9	100.0
Referrals to community services	28.4	35.1	36.6	100.1
Counseling	29.9	30.4	39.7	100.0
Food	41.8	31.3	26.9	100.0
Discharge plan	23.3	12.9	63.9	100.1
Bill of Rights	13.3	37.6	49.0	99.9
Grievance/staff	44.3	37.4	18.2	99.9
Grievance/medical	34.3	36.9	28.8	100.0
Grievance/patient care	48.0	36.8	15.2	100.0
Advocate/patients	49.5	35.2	15.2	99.9
Advocate/community groups	13.7	18.8	67.5	100.0
Data channeling	52.3	36.4	11.2	99.9
Monitors malpractice	15.4	28.4	56.3	100.1
Identifies malpractice policies	12.2	28.3	59.5	100.0
Change hospital rules	15.1	50.5	34.4	100.0
Fee information	32.7	34.6	32.7	100.0
Recommend adjustment of bill	24.8	29.1	46.1	100.0
Adjusts bill	9.8	5.4	84.8	100.0
Represents account	13.9	7.5	78.6	100.0
Orientation	26.9	15.9	57.2	100.0
Education	16.1	22.0	62.0	100.1

patient representative programs, although they may be important components of a few specialized programs.

The 28 activities were then grouped together by means of a factor analysis to determine whether types or "profiles" of patient representative programs could be identified. Four patterns emerged that seem to represent four separate types of programs, although none of them was completely "pure" nor did they perform mutually exclusive activities. Of these four types of programs, all but the Financial Services program provide significant prototypes which can be replicated in a variety of hospitals.

About half of the programs in the study were classified as "Grievance," a name attached to the type of program in which a patient representative investigated complaints from patients, channeled information about those complaints to appropriate departments, and responded to grievances of patients about the care they received from the medical and other hospital staff. Some of the programs had, in addition, a monitoring role in patient care problems in which there was the potential for malpractice suits.

The second type of program, called "Patient Services," was less prevalent in the study group: 25 percent of the sample. Patient representatives in this type of program performed some of the services that are often, although not exclusively, associated with social workers in hospitals. Patient representatives referred patients to community facilities, made discharge plans, and provided counseling services. They also secured transportation and translators when necessary and provided information to community groups about the hospital.

The third type of program, named "Hospitality Services" was less distinct in its profile of activities. Patient representatives of this type welcomed patients upon admission, arranged for television rentals, parking permits, beautician appointments, and so forth, and in other ways attended to amenities that were not the first priority of other hospital staff. They also provided information about the hospital to patients and their families and responded to complaints about food and housekeeping services. The hospitality services were the least well defined of the types of programs since providing information and responding to food and housekeeping complaints were activities that the grievance and patient services programs also performed. The distinguishing set of characteristics that separated hospitality programs from others was the core courtesy services. When these predominated, the program was considered to belong to the hospitality type.

A fourth type of program called "Financial Services" also emerged in the factor analysis, and 17 percent of the hospitals studied had programs of this type. Financial services programs focused largely on the hospital's financial relations with patients. A financial officer was designated to whom patients could direct all inquiries and complaints about bills, insurance, and other possible reimbursements. These programs had quite different goals and activities than the other types of patient representative programs and were connected with them principally by a common name rather than a generic purpose or function.

Seven Case Studies of Patient Representative Programs

The Survey of Patient Representatives Study illustrated these profiles of patient representative programs with descriptions of seven hospital programs. In each hospital the circumstances under which the patient representative program was introduced were explored through tape-recorded interviews with hospital staff members. Although all of the programs had unique beginnings, some common experiences in their development could be identified. All began out of a recognition of need by at least one segment of the hospital system in response to a group of problems which were perceived as not being resolvable by assignment to an already existing department or service. In most hospitals programs were developed to deal with problems or gaps in service that were interdepartmental in scope. Some programs were established as a result of pressure from groups or individuals outside of the boundaries of the hospital system while others came as a result of initiatives from within. The acceptance of patient representative programs into the hospital structure often had political implications, either at the level of the relationship between the hospital and the community or the relationship between various groups within the hospital.

In addition to these similarities, each program had unique characteristics. To a certain extent, the differences in programs were related to the history of how and by whom the program was formulated, as well as by such factors as the traditions of the hospital and its characteristic ways of handling problems.

Adams General Hospital—A Patient Services Program *

At Adams General, a 600-bed, prestigious, voluntary teaching hospital with a tradition of an active involvement with the community, the proposal for a patient representative program for the emergency room came from their Community Advisory Board. While the problems in the emergency room at Adams had been identified and documented over and over again by various individuals and departments within the hospital

---

*The names of the hospitals are fictitious and the number of beds has been rounded off to increase confidentiality.

structure, it continued to be a trouble spot for the hospital board and staff and a source of frustration to patients and those who accompanied them. One member of the social work staff described the situation in the emergency room at that time:

> . . . the emergency room, the waiting room, it was a jungle, a dangerous place . . . feared and disliked . . . everything negative . . . There were incidents. Staff members were attacked verbally and literally.

The patients experienced long waiting periods in cramped, drab surroundings. Their frustrations were exacerbated by an overworked staff who did not or could not take the time to provide appropriate information either to the patients or to their waiting families once the patients were taken in for examination or treatment.

The hospital officially defined the problem in terms of inadequate resources: staff, money, and space. Informally, however, it was defined by some members of the staff as a classical conflict between the teaching and service functions of the hospital. Residents and interns carried responsibility for most of the work of the emergency room, and it was an important teaching resource for them. The appointment of a full-time paid physician to be in charge of the residents and the emergency room would, in the opinion of some of the staff, have improved service. However, this was strongly resisted by some of the most powerful medical chiefs of service in the hospital because it would reduce their hegemony over the teaching function.

The social work department recognized the critical need of the emergency room population for social work services, and assigned two shifts of social workers there so that there was coverage from 8:00 A.M. until midnight. It also deployed a number of trained volunteers to work in that area. Yet there continued to be much patient dissatisfaction with the service. The nursing department was disturbed by the disruptive behavior of patients and their families because it distracted nurses from their appropriate duties. They depended on security officers as the chief means of maintaining order and safety.

The community, through its Community Advisory Board, defined the situation in the emergency room in different terms. They saw the problems in terms of poor communication between the staff and patients and their families. They felt that if there were a better flow of information between them some of the frustration on both sides could be avoided. They proposed a patient representative program which would use community volunteers as major bridging persons to facilitate the flow of information.

The Community Advisory Board at Adams had a long tradition of active involvement with the hospital and occupied a position of considerable influence with them. The departments of social work, nursing, and administration sent representatives to each of the advisory board meetings, and a sense of accountability to the community was evident in all the attitudes of those interviewed at Adams. This attitude was summed up by a comment from their administrator:

> The hospital has served the community for (many) years . . . There tends to be the feeling that it is our job. Consequently, 'demands' made by the community do not upset this hospital . . . it feels that's what it is supposed to be doing anyhow.

Therefore, when the Community Advisory Board prepared a proposal for a patient representative program for the emergency room, it was not experienced by the hospital as adversary or intrusive. While some hospital personnel had reservations about the *idea* of a patient representative program per se, the fact that it emanated from the community did not seem to stir up opposition. In fact, the hospital helped the board write a proposal for a grant to fund the project, and assisted it in many ways in trying to get the project funded. Eventually a philanthropic fund of a private corporation provided a grant, and the program went into operation shortly afterward.

Davis Hospital Center—A Grievance Program

The Davis Hospital Center, a 1,000-bed public teaching hospital, also developed a patient representative program partially on the initiative of outside community pressure. The hospital was going through a period in which the quality of service was being severely threatened by reductions in funding, curtailment of staff to dangerous levels, shortage of essential supplies, threats from unions, and other serious problems common to public hospitals in the 1970s.

Community dissatisfaction was vocal and was expressed through the Community Advisory Board and its subcommittee, the Patient Care Committee. The Patient Care Committee was inundated with complaints and requests from community members for help in seeking redress for problems they were encountering in the hospital. At first, the committee tried to respond individually to the requests of its constituents and to pursue each complaint with the appropriate department. However, it was evident that it did not have either the capability or the resources for effective intervention within the hospital system. It identified the need for a structure within the hospital to which it could bring the community's complaints and requests for information. It wanted the hospital to designate a specific person who would be able to respond to complaints and to act as an advocate for patients in all of the departments and services of the hospital. It expected that while it would no longer directly intervene for its constituents, the designated person would be accountable to it.

While the committee did not seek outside funding as a means of control, it expected to exercise a considerable amount of informal power, based not only upon the legally mandated relationship between public hospitals and Community Advisory Boards, but also upon the amount of pressure that they could exert in a time when all of the public hospitals were in a position of vulnerability in relation to community groups. There was considerable responsiveness by the administration of the hospital to the Patient Care Committee's demand. Davis already had a small patient relations program, staffed by several clerical-level employees. This formed the nucleus for the new program which was given status and power by the appointment of a patient representative, approved by the Community Advisory Board, at the rank of associate director of the hospital. The patient representative was specifically designated as a permanent liaison to the Patient Care Committee and was expected to be responsive to it.

In contrast to Adams Hospital, the relationship between the patient representative and the Patient Care Committee at Davis has often been problematic. Committee members are sometimes considered by the patient representative to be intrusive, self-seeking, and dominated by personal politics.

> It's a burden . . . two kinds of people make up the committee. Those who are politically interested . . . politically motivated, and those who are interested in getting service for themselves.

At the beginning, the patient representative often had to take steps to limit the committee members and to redefine their appropriate stance as a committee. She saw herself as being in a position to make judgments about whether complaints from the community were justified and to advocate for them only when appropriate. She discouraged their direct interference on behalf of individual community members. In spite of these problems, however, the committee has continued to support the patient representative and the program, and to encourage its growth.

Barry Hospital—A Patient Services Program

At Barry Hospital the initiative for the patient representative program also came from outside the regular hospital hierarchy. In this case, the initiative came not from a community group or advisory board, but from a member of the hospital's auxiliary board who functioned as a volunteer in the hospital. The volunteer worked in the surgical waiting room where her task was to facilitate messages from surgeons to relatives of patients who were awaiting the outcome of surgery. Her contacts with relatives of patients convinced her and a number of other auxiliary members that there was a need for a program that advocated for patients and helped them to deal more effectively with the professional bureaucracy of the hospital.

Their proposal to the hospital director for a patient representative program was favorably received. However, when the idea was presented to the heads of the medical and administrative staffs of the hospital, there was considerable opposition. Both the auxiliary board members and the program they proposed were perceived as adversary in approach and hostile to the professional and nonprofessional hospital staff. Nevertheless, the program was established. An important factor favoring its establishment was that the volunteers had considerable influence of a social and kinship nature with members of the hospital board of directors. It was their pressure that prevailed; most staff considered it politically unwise to fight against a proposal supported by the board of directors. The costs of the all-volunteer program were carried by the auxiliary board, and the hospital made almost no financial commitment. There continued to be very little sanction from most of the hospital professional staff as evidenced by the fact that the program began on only one medical inpatient ward without formal announcement or introduction of it or of the patient representative to the staff.

Farwell Hospital Center—A Grievance Program

In contrast to the first three hospitals, the patient representative program at Farwell Hospital was initiated from within the hospital bureaucratic structure. In this hospital, the program was proposed as a part of the social work department's activities. It began in the outpatient clinics and emergency room, and its goals were to provide outreach, information and referral, and advocacy to patients as well as data collection and feedback to the hospital on problems in the use of outpatient services. The program was modeled after the idea of the Neighborhood Information Centers in England in that it was perceived to be a structure to deal with unpredictable dysfunctions or obstructions in service rather than a provider of direct service.[4]

Farwell, a 1,200-bed, teaching, voluntary medical center was undergoing many changes when the patient representative program was conceived. It was growing in size and becoming more complex because of the addition of a medical school to its facilities. In addition, its outpatient department was experiencing a change in patient population. With the advent of Medicare and Medicaid there was increased pressure for the utilization of Farwell's clinic facilities by minority group residents of the immediate neighborhood. The social work department, as part of the Community Medicine Division, proposed the establishment of a patient representative program. The program was intended to help community residents who, through language difficulties or other problems, were experiencing obstacles of access or use of clinic or emergency room facilities. Then, on the basis of the data collected from patients' complaints or problems with the hospital, it was to make recommendations about ways to deal with the system dysfunction it encountered. The program had considerable hospital support, and after a planning phase of six months it went into operation.

Caroline Hospital—A Hospitality Program

Caroline Hospital, a 600-bed community hospital with a very limited teaching function, also established its patient representative program as a result of initiative from within the hospital structure. In this case, it was hospital administration that formulated and supported the program. While earlier there was a public relations and fundraising courtesy program, which directed its services toward wealthy private patients in the hospital, the reorganized patient representative program was broadened to include all inpatients. The impetus for the development of the program came from the hospital administrator's perception of a need for an individual on staff who was not directly responsible for any direct service for patients and, therefore, could be responsive to patient complaints about problems encountered in the hospital. He saw all other hospital personnel as having specific role responsibilities which they pursued either directly or indirectly with patients. He wanted to have someone whose role could be exclusively devoted to attending to patient satisfaction. A former volunteer who had been trained by the social work department of the hospital was hired for the new program, partially because she was a person with skills in working with patients and because she knew the hospital system.

Emerson Hospital—A Grievance Program

The patient representative program in Emerson Hospital, a 1,400-bed prestigious voluntary hospital, was initiated by the director of the hospital. He described its beginnings:

> We were aware of the fact that there were a lot of questions raised by patients and families, or by the staff in relation to patients . . . questions that somehow did not fit neatly into some box . . . So there always were a certain number of these problems that just seemed to be around, and (always the question was) who should be the individual to tackle that problem . . . By virtue of the fact that in many instances it was not obvious

that the problem could be neatly slotted into the administrative hierarchy, the idea developed that what we probably needed was an individual who did not belong to any department, but who could move readily around the institution, to deal with the amazing diversity of problems, some financial, some social, some dealing with the professional staff . . . doctors and nurses . . . you name it . . . across the board kinds of problems.

The director established the patient representative program as a direct adjunct to his own office, and he saw it as an important administrative mechanism that would be responsive to patient care problems. Of the seven hospital programs investigated, this patient representative program had the highest level of hospital commitment. It not only had been initiated by the director but the program had the support of the board of trustees of the hospital as well as medical board. It was carefully introduced to each of the departments and service areas with the highly visible support of the director of the hospital.

Guardian Hospital—A Hospitality Program

Guardian Hospital's patient representative program had an entirely different beginning. Guardian is a 200-bed voluntary church operated (Catholic) exurban nonteaching hospital. The patient representative program developed because of the chaplain's need for someone to tend to patients' complaints about food, housekeeping, and other nonmedical care problems as well as to assist him with the provision of religious support to families and patients. A Catholic Sister was appointed to the position and the program was begun with the clear understanding that its scope would be limited to nonmedical matters. As the patient representative described it:

I try to answer questions within my capacity. I'll never answer questions about nursing care or doctors' problems . . . If it's something to do with doctors, I'll say, '*that* you will have to take up with the doctor personally.'

This clear definition was reechoed by the hospital administrator:

I see it as a patient representative thing . . . liaison . . . sometimes you don't see the trees for the forest . . . You (the patient) don't like something that is going on . . . When it is outlined, we can do something about it. But not so as you get into a consumer representative . . . The board would never agree to that!

Because the program was established as part of the religious structure of the hospital and because of its unobtrusive scope, there was virtually no opposition to it by the top level of the hospital staff.

*The Further Development of the Patient Representative Program in
Each Hospital*

While the establishment of patient representative programs in each
of the seven hospitals took a different course, and met with varying degrees
of acceptance by the upper echelons of the hospital administrative and
medical staff, they were invariably regarded with hostility and distrust at
the level of line workers. Some reluctance could have been expected on the
part of established occupational groups to having to share functions or
responsibilities they viewed as within their own domain. Resistance to
change, while often irrationally expressed, was very real and was based on
the fear of loss of autonomy, prestige and status, positive regard from
patients, and, ultimately, loss of job. Nurses, social workers, and other
hospital staff expressed varying degrees of anger at the introduction of the
new program, fearing that the patient representative might get in the way,
interfere with established practices, or take the side of patients against
them. While all of these sentiments were expressed at the beginning in each
program, the problems were resolved in different ways.

At Adams, where the patient representative program is confined to
the emergency room, the nursing supervisor tried to insure that the staff
understood the new program by holding formal meetings with supervisory
nursing personnel. In spite of careful preparation there were problems
between nurses and patient representatives. At first, the nurses' complaints
centered around the issue that the patient representatives were all volunteers. The nurses questioned the fact that volunteers would have access to
patients' medical charts. The nurses worried about the confidential information in the chart as well as the inability of the volunteer to correctly
interpret medical information to patients' families. Underlying this was a
feeling on the part of some of the nurses that patient representatives were
undermining their relationship with patients.

> The patient advocate is making me look like the bad guy. She talks to the
> patient and sympathizes.

Another underlying source of resentment was the feeling of nurses that the
patient representative was monitoring their behavior. An issue of professional status was involved. The nurses resented that a lay person, especially a volunteer, should have them under surveillance. "She's always
looking over my shoulder," was a common complaint.

Other staff members also had problems with the role of the patient
representative. It infringed on the former responsibilities of the emergency
room registrar and triage clerk. These staff members complained that the
patient representative was getting in the way and, in addition, that the
latter was not performing adequately the tasks that formerly belonged to
them. There was also a clash with several of the emergency room social

workers. One feared that the patient representative would try to exercise authority over her. Another felt that her professional work with patients was being interfered with. She spoke about a problem she faced in her work with a group of patients where her goal was to mobilize the anger of members of the group so as to help them with their depressions. She felt that the patient representative was being overly solicitous of patients, which reduced the effectiveness of what the social worker was trying to do.

The initial defensiveness and conflict at Adams gradually subsided. At one level, the improvement came because a series of meetings were held with the patient representative and the emergency room staff in which problems were aired and roles were more clearly defined. At another level, both the nurses and social workers began to see benefits for them in the presence of the program in the hospital. The waiting room was quieter. There were fewer complaints and fewer disruptions. The social worker came to realize that, in spite of problems, the presence of the patient representative was helpful to her. It was not necessary for her or the nurse to be called into the waiting room so often to deal with angry patients or families, and so she had more time to devote to other aspects of her work.

The experience at Davis was similar. The nurses feared loss of autonomy and were afraid of being spied upon. They felt that the patient representative would always side with patients. They worried that if the patient representative (who was also an associate director of the hospital) would find them at fault, it might jeopardize their jobs.

Resentment by the social workers was based on some of the same feelings. The line social workers worried that the patient representative might take over their jobs. They were threatened by the apparent and real power that the patient representative possessed and her capacity to make quick decisions without consultation. The resentment also came from the fact that many of the social workers had identified some of the same patient care problems the patient representative was finding, but could never get the administrative staff to respond to their complaints or to make changes. The patient representative was able to get things accomplished very quickly and effectively.

Again, as at Adams, after a period of time the relationships between the patient representative and the other staff at Davis improved. The same dynamic of mutuality developed, and the staff began to see the value to them of the patient representative. As the director of social work said:

> What started happening was that the social workers came across patients in the hospital or clinic . . . patients with problems that they could not help to solve. They recognized that this was just the kind of thing that if they got the advocate involved in, could get done. And vice versa, the patient advocate was being inundated with problems that she knew could be handled by social service and she was glad to refer them. So on the bottom level, on a case by case basis, we worked things out. We needed each other.

> We find now that nothing terrible will happen if we share a problem. I
> don't think we are afraid of each other any more. We use each other: the
> flavor of the relationship has changed.

In Farwell, where the patient representative program was initiated by
the social work department, there was resistance to the program from an
additional source. The administrator in charge of all of the outpatient
clinics thought that the program should be under his jurisdiction and since
it was not he objected to its existence. The problem was solved only when
the administrator went on to a new job. Some conflict also arose at the
beginning of the program with the nurses. They felt that the patient
representative was "a spying operation." It took time for them to develop
trust. Even in the social work department, in which the patient representative program was located, there was initial resistance and conflict. Some
of the social workers thought that the patient representative was defining
problems that were really more centrally related to the emotional problems of the patient than a result of system dysfunction. The patient representative on her part thought that social workers sometimes "dumped" on
her problems they should really have handled themselves. In this hospital,
as in the others, there was a gradual change in attitude toward the program as it demonstrated its value to the various groups of professionals.

The patient representative at Emerson saw the gradual dissolution of
resistance to her program as being a result of the great effort she made to
be helpful to the staff. She found that she gained acceptance as she did
things for the staff that either made their jobs easier or alleviated a personal or professional problem they were having.

> The staff learned that I was not out to hang their dirty wash in public, or
> to do their jobs. I would go out of my way to get things done for the
> nursing staff that they couldn't get done by themselves. For example,
> because I knew the engineer, I became a miracle worker, I could get things
> done that no one else could.

Resistance at this hospital also came from physicians. Because of the
patient representative's position as assistant to the director, and because
she became involved in patient care problems involving possible medical
malpractice, the physicians were finding themselves accountable to a nonmedical person in a way that they had not previously experienced. A status
issue developed; some of the physicians became openly angry and resistive
to the program and to the patient representative. Again, the acceptance
of the program by the physicians took place gradually and often in response to incidents in which the patient representative would expedite
things which the doctors were not able to accomplish in the hospital
system by themselves.

The patient representatives in both Emerson and Farwell were quite
conscious of the use of professional favor-giving as a means of reducing
distrust and resistance. However, they realized that it was a double-edged

tool. On the one hand, it improved relationships and gained acceptance for the program; on the other, it put them in a position of performing activities that might really be the function and responsibility of other professional or occupational groups. The issue became one of guarding against the manipulativeness of other staff while still maintaining a stance of being useful to them.

At Barry General Hospital, a different approach was necessary. Demonstrating usefulness was not enough. The opposition to the patient representative program was quite deep-seated and was not confined to line level workers. Because of ongoing problems, the medical director at Barry created a special committee on patient care, which met regularly with representatives of the physician group, social work, nursing, administration, and the patient representative in an attempt to lower the level of mutual suspicion. In the opinion of the director of social work, the committee did little to improve patient care in the hospital, but it did serve as an excellent instrument of training for the patient representative. The latter began to be aware of some of the problems of the hospital and its professionals in delivering services. In effect she was coopted into the system, and her adversary, antiprofessional stance was partially vitiated. However, the staff has remained more or less unaccepting of the program, even though the patient representative continues to try to work through problems as they occur.

In the church-operated Guardian Hospital there was minor opposition even among the nurses. As the director of nursing said,

> At first there were times when there was a cardiac arrest when she (the patient representative) was getting in the way of people actually performing their work . . . She herself didn't realize it. We had to talk to her. But these things got straightened out. Now we have come full swing. If the patient representative does not show when there is a cardiac arrest, the nurses have her paged. She is so very good with families, particularly in the waiting area of the emergency room.

The Process of Institutionalization of the Patient Representative Programs in the Seven Hospitals

The development of patient representative programs was a result of two ongoing processes of accommodation. The first was the beginning adaptation of the hospital system to the introduction of a new program and occupational group as described above. The second was the process of change within the patient representative program so as to fit into the institutional context. Four elements of development were examined: changes in the scope of activities of the patient representative programs, extent of their coverage, staffing, and referral patterns. While no cause and effect connections should be made on the basis of such limited evidence, these patterns of change of the patient representative programs seemed to be associated with at least three critical elements: the pattern of funding, their location in the organizational hierarchy, and the flexibility of their goals.

The method of funding seemed to be an indication of the level of institutional commitment to the program. Organizations usually try to bring a program important to its functioning under its control by including it within its budget.[5] Two out of the seven patient representative programs studied were initially financed by grants awarded by outside agencies, and the programs thus had power connections outside of the direct administrative control of the hospital. Both of these programs had a low level of change. However, while the absence of financing by the hospital seemed to be associated with minimal change of the patient representative programs, hospital funding alone did not seem to be enough to ensure growth. Thus, while it is true that the programs with the highest or medium change levels were all funded by the hospitals themselves, one program that remained virtually unchanged was also so funded.

Another element that seemed to be important in how the patient representative program fared was the auspices or location within the organizational structure that it occupied. The two programs that have changed most dramatically, both grievance programs, have been those in which the patient representatives reported directly to the highest corporate administrative officers of the hospitals. Each had, by virtue of the position in the organizational structure, a high level of power, either ascribed or delegated. The two programs with departmental status, or whose patient representative reported to the second or third level of the administrative hierarchy, had a medium level of change. The other three, those with a low change rate, reported to officers even lower in the structure.

The third factor that seemed to affect the growth of the patient representative program was whether the goals enunciated at the beginning of the program were flexible enough to allow for change. The two programs that had the most specific statement of goals were initially financed by grants. It is not clear whether the process of proposal-writing forced an articulation of goals that locked in the programs or whether the combination of sharply defined goals and low institutional commitment were operating together.

High Change Programs

The patient representative program at Emerson was an example of a unit with a high growth and change level. Administratively, the patient representative had the title of assistant to the director of the hospital and was responsible directly to him. Institutional sanction for the program was very high and funding came directly from the hospital's administrative budget. While the patient representative had no formal power attached to her office, she had a high level of delegated as well as informal power.

When the program was initiated the goals of the program were intentionally kept flexible. The director of the hospital described the goal setting process:

> I didn't sit down with a piece of paper and draw up a job description. I didn't *want* to precisely define what the activities would be or assign her to any specific committees. It turned into a tailor-made job. It could have stopped at a patient service level, and that would have been fine, but she had interests that met other institutional needs. So the program evolved. That's what I had in mind.

The patient representative at Emerson described the growth of the scope of activities of the program from her point of view:

> When I started, I dealt with personal service problems. I was like a paid volunteer, visiting people. I used to make rounds to the private patients . . . a floor a day, and I would talk to patients. I dealt with housekeeping problems, scheduling problems and minor billing. I never got involved in writeoffs (of bills) or making recommendations for reductions (in fees) . . . I certainly never dreamt . . . never even heard the word malpractice. Then when I got more comfortable in talking to patients and was able to gear my interviewing skills to be more than superficial, I began to get into patient care problems, mostly complaints about nursing care . . . Eventually, I got into more serious problems; first, attitudes of doctors, then complaints about their competency or ineptitude. Now I deal with claims investigations and risk management . . . the malpractice cases. (Much of it is) the negotiation with the patients to try to get something resolved without any of us having to go to court. My staff still keep up with some of the simpler patient care problems . . . some of the things that we started to do at the beginning, we still do them.

Other changes took place in the program as it grew. Its scope of coverage enlarged. While at first it was directed toward private patients in one 200-bed section of the hospital, it later covered all parts of the hospital, both inpatient and outpatient, and served all patients regardless of their form of payment. It also offered limited service to employees and house staff. The staff of the program has grown to three full-time workers. While volunteers have been used from time to time, they have been involved in selected ways, dealing mostly with casefinding. Almost all of the patients served by the program are currently based on referrals, both from the staff and from patients, and the practice of making patient rounds is no longer generally carried on.

Thus, the program at Emerson has changed in four major components: scope of activities, scope of coverage, staffing, and referral patterns. It evolved from a small hospitality program for private patients into a grievance program with a high level of responsibility and authority for solving all kinds of problems about patient care. While part of the program still responds to the less complex complaints of individual patients, the person in charge of the program is mostly concerned with systems change and risk management activities.

The patient representative program at Davis Hospital is the other example of a program with a high level of growth or change. While the initial idea of creating a patient representative program came from the Community Board, there was considerable institutional commitment to the project. Funds were provided from the hospital budget, and the patient representative was given considerable formal power by virtue of her title as associate director of the hospital. The goals of the program were not clearly enunciated at the beginning, but since the patient representative had both institutional commitment and power, she was able to expand the program in all areas. It grew in scope, coverage, and changed in staffing patterns and method of referrals. The patient representative described its expansion of activities and scope as follows:

> What has happened is that we started out with a *Patient's Bill of Rights,* trying to help patients get good care, and we have just ballooned. It is like somebody put too much baking power in a biscuit and it's gotten bigger and bigger. And the problems are getting worse because of cutbacks in the hospital budget and staff. The morale (of the staff) is low and attitudes are bad. The problems are unending. I have taken over the child abuse program in the hospital. I testify in court on behalf of the hospital and deal with the press. I am on long-range beeper 24 hours a day, seven days a week, and when I leave the range of the beeper, I have to give it to someone else. Once, I was called in because two men took over a ward. It was me that they called to deal with it. They (the men) took 13 hostages and threatened that they had bombs. There is no end to the trouble.

Besides changes in scope of activities and coverage of the program, the patient representative at Davis has made other unique changes in the staffing pattern of the program. In addition to increasing the paid staff to three full-time workers, the program has begun to use the services of a physician who works as a volunteer. A person of considerable prestige in the medical world and an emeritus dean of a medical school, he acts as a consultant to the patient representative program, reviewing complaints about medical care provided by the hospital. At first, the patient representative was suspicious of his offer to serve as a volunteer as she thought he might be defensive of the medical establishment, but now she values his services highly and uses them to good effect in exploring complaints with medical components and in communicating with the medical staff of the hospital.

Thus Davis began as a grievance and information program for responding to complaints from community residents about patient care problems. However, it has developed into a major hospital program with responsibility and authority for "trouble shooting" about a wide variety of patient care and public relations problems.

Medium Change Programs

The patient representative program at Farwell Hospital evolved along somewhat different lines, and its rate of change has been moderate. In contrast to Davis and Emerson, where the patient representative reports to the highest corporate officer in the hospital, at Farwell she reports to the third level of authority and so has less formal or informal power. However, since she does report to the director of social work and, most recently, the director of nursing, both of whom are voting members of the medical board of the hospital, there is access through them to the highest level of decision-making. In her own right the patient representative is a member of a number of lesser decision-making committees in the hospital which allows her to directly raise important patient care issues. She also has considerable personal prestige and freedom of movement throughout the hospital in investigating patient complaints and gathering data.

The program began with two clearly defined goals: removing obstacles to patient care and identifying system dysfunction. As the program became firmly established, the latter goal gained in importance. The patient representative observed that

> We knew we would never have enough patient representatives to take care of all of the people with problems. We very consciously used the patient problems with which we were dealing to try to make the system more responsive to patient needs. As the hospital has grown larger, we have changed our focus. We have kept up the very personalized responsiveness to patients, but there has been an expansion of the role of change agent.

Other changes that have taken place in the patient representative program at Farwell have been in the expansion of coverage and scope of activities as well as staffing patterns. The original program, which covered only the outpatient and emergency room services, was being extended to the inpatient service at the time of the study. A small personal service and courtesy program for inpatients that had been functioning as a separate entity was incorporated into an enlarged patient representative program. The scope of activities of the program was also enlarged because of the kind of services provided to inpatients. The number of staff members increased to three workers and one half-time worker and more volunteers were being selectively assigned to some special tasks.

Farwell's program thus has grown largely as a result of changing from an outpatient to a combined outpatient and inpatient program. It started out as a grievance program and remains so, but more emphasis is now being placed on the systems change aspects of the program than at the beginning.

The other patient representative program with a medium level of growth or change was Caroline. Caroline's patient representative program is a hospital-funded program. Its goals were somewhat nebulous at the time the program started. In contrast to Emerson, however, the openness of the goals has not led to expansion of the program to any considerable extent. In terms of organizational location, the program moved from a staff position as part of administration to full departmental status at the same level as the social work and nursing departments. This has given the patient representative more formal power as she now has access to those decision-making committees that include heads of departments.

The program at Caroline has changed very little in terms of scope of activities and only moderately in terms of coverage. It was initiated as a hospitality inpatient program responding to patient complaints about housekeeping, nursing care, and so forth, and has continued along these lines. Its method of referral is still largely by making rounds of new patients who have been admitted each day. Its philosophy has consistently been to alleviate problems of patients on a case-by-case basis, but does not emphasize activities of feedback or system change to the same extent as some of the other programs described.

The one major area in which there has been change in the program at Caroline has been in its staffing pattern. There are now two paid patient representatives whose service has been augmented by eight well-trained volunteers, each of whom spends several days a week working in the program. In the opinion of the administrator of the hospital, the inclusion of volunteers in the program has increased not only the amount of service that could be offered to patients, but also the program's prestige in the hospital. This is because most of the volunteers are in the same social circle or kinship network as members of the board of trustees.

Thus, the major changes in the program at Caroline have been an expansion of staff and an increase in formal power based on its elevation to departmental status. However, little change has occurred in scope of activities. While the goals of the program were loosely formulated there was a high level of consensus about its function, and there has been no major thrust to change the program or increase its activities within the hospital.

Low Change Programs

The patient representative program at Barry has evidenced relatively little growth or change. The program had a very low level of hospital commitment, and at the time it was studied was not yet well accepted by the hospital staff. It continued to be considered a burden by them rather than contributory to patient care. However, because of the informal power of the individuals who began the program and funded it, the patient representative program continued to function.

The one area of change in the program at Barry was in its staffing pattern. In contrast to the program at Caroline which started with a paid patient representative and then enlarged its scope by the addition of a volunteer staff, Barry's program started with volunteers and only later added a paid patient representative. The volunteers who originally began the program recognized that they could cover only a limited number of service areas and eventually proposed that a paid worker be hired who would conduct the patient representative program on an ongoing basis and who would enlarge the scope of its coverage. The paid worker further augmented her staff by the use of undergraduate students who wanted some field work experience in a hospital as part of their education. The patient representative coordinated their work and provided them with supervision. The staff thus consists of a mix of volunteer auxiliary board members who initiated the program, a paid staff member, and the student group. This has allowed for an expansion in the number of inpatient services covered by the program. There have been no major changes in the scope of activities or method of referrals. It started as a personal service program and has continued along the same lines.

The patient representative program at Adams, another low growth program, has also remained fairly stable with few changes. The level of institutional commitment to the program is not totally clear. While the hospital administrator stated that if funding of the program were not renewed from the outside, the hospital would pick up the costs of the program in its own budget, its reason for doing so would relate more to the unwillingness to offend the Community Advisory Board than from the commitment to the idea of a patient representative. The patient representative reports to a third-level corporate officer in the hospital administrative structure and has little formal power. She does derive some power from the support of the Community Advisory Board and, while she can do little to coerce, she is often deferred to in order to avoid friction with the community. Begun as an emergency room program with trained volunteers and one paid person, it has made no significant changes in its staffing patterns, scope of activities, referrals, or coverage. While the proposal that funded the project stipulated that the scope of coverage would eventually be expanded to include outpatient clinic services, this has not yet taken place, and the program remains small and encapsulated.

The patient representative program at Guardian Hospital has evidenced the least change of all of the hospitals studied. While it is a program that is funded by the hospital, it has almost no power and its goals are quite restricted. The Sister who has been in charge of the program has taken on additional religious responsibilities, giving communion to those patients who wish it and assisting the chaplain in other religious tasks. However, the program continues to adhere to a philosophy of attending to complaints about the nonmedical problems of patients and of offering solace and comfort to the ill and their families.

In summary, there has been a range of patterns of evolution of the patient representative programs within each of the seven hospitals. Some of the programs have had a remarkable period of growth in times when hospitals are being forced to cut budgets fairly drastically. The fate of each program seems to be somewhat idiosyncratic, although the most important variables in the expansion of the programs studied seemed to be the power of the constituency that initiated the program and the commitment of hospital administration to it.

Characteristics of the Patient Representatives in the Programs in the Seven Hospitals

The further question of whether there was any association between the characteristics of the person hired to direct the patient representative program and how they developed remains unclear. In five out of the seven hospitals, the first person hired to fill the position of patient representative was still the incumbent at the time of the study. The sex, age, ethnic group, and educational or vocational background of each incumbent patient representative was examined. In general, while it was evident that these or other attributes of the patient representative might have contributed in some way to how the program developed, there was little objective evidence for confirmation. The form that the programs took seems to be multidetermined, and the contribution of the personal characteristics of the patient representative is difficult to measure. Nevertheless, it is interesting to note their characteristics to illustrate that they constituted a group with a range of educational and vocational backgrounds as well as a variety of special skills which they brought to their new jobs.

The patient representative at Adams Hospital was a social worker with a master of social work degree and over 10 years of experience. She functioned as a community organizer for the hospital prior to her appointment as a patient representative. In that position, she was considered part of hospital administration, and was not under the jurisdiction of the regular social work department. She had many political contacts, was active in local community organizations, and represented the hospital on a number of health planning boards. She was knowledgeable about the workings of the hospital, and when the proposal of the Community Advisory Board of the hospital was funded, she was the natural choice of both the community and hospital administration.

The patient representative at Emerson was completing a health planning degree (MPA) in a school of public administration at the time of the study. She also had a bachelor of science degree in nursing. She was employed at Emerson as a nurse until she became ill, and then spent some time as a patient in another hospital. This gave her an added perspective about patient care. At a social occasion, she got into a conversation with the director of the hospital and told him some of her ideas about how patient care could be improved. He had been considering the creation of a patient representative program and later offered her the job.

The patient representative at Farwell Hospital was the only other incumbent in the study with a baccalaureate. She had been working in the hospital in an administrative position prior to her appointment as a patient representative. She knew the hospital quite well and was highly regarded by the social work staff with whom she had worked closely. She was hired by the director of social work, in whose department the patient representative program was located.

At Davis Hospital, the patient representative was hired with the approval of the Community Advisory Board as well as the hospital. She had no college degree but had extensive experience in handling consumer complaints. She had been an assistant to the mayor of a large city and, among other things, had been responsible for responding to citizen complaints about government agencies. While she did not then have the title of ombudsman, she functioned informally in that role. With a change of city administration, she was looking for a new position. Her experience in handling consumer complaints, her reputation for being able to effectively accomplish tasks in spite of red tape, and her political connections were influential in her selection as patient representative.

At Barry, the patient representative had been at her present job for over a year. Prior to her incumbency, the program had been staffed by two volunteers. She had no baccalaureate, but had prior experience as a patient representative in another hospital. It was this attribute that was important in her being hired for the job at Barry.

The patient representative at Caroline also had no baccalaureate, but had been a volunteer at the hospital prior to being hired for the job. The job became vacant when the first incumbent decided to go to graduate school. At that time the administrator who was in charge of the program looked specifically for someone who was older, who knew the hospital, and who could supervise a volunteer program of patient representatives.

The woman who was the patient representative at Guardian was a nun who had no college degree. She had been assigned to her hospital, which is church operated, for over 30 years, functioning first as a teacher for long-term hospitalized children and then as an administrator for an outpatient clinic. She received her current assignment when the hospital chaplain, a Catholic priest, suggested that a patient representative program be established. She was appointed by the Mother Superior on the basis of her attributes as a gentle, empathic person who could relate to the spiritual needs of the patients as well as to their personal complaints. She knew the hospital extremely well and was highly regarded by the staff.

Thus in five of the seven programs the patient representatives had worked at their hospitals in either paid or unpaid positions before being hired for their present jobs. They had a high degree of familiarity with the hospital, and this was an important asset in their new jobs. The two patient representatives who were hired from outside the hospital both brought relevant experience to the jobs which in some way compensated for their lack of knowledge of the hospital.

In summary, while the programs themselves and the hospitals in which they were established are not intended to be prototypical or representative of the range that exists in the United States, they do provide some illuminating data. It is quite evident that each of the programs was unique in the way it was founded and in the course of its development. While some activities were performed by all of them, each program was distinctive in its form and function. All were relatively new at the time they were investigated and were in the process of evolution. It is not clear whether patient representative programs at some future time will become less diverse in purpose and organizational form with a more explicitly conceptualized and well-accepted purpose and function.

References

1. Society of Patient Representatives. "A Descriptive Definition." Chicago (mimeographed, undated).
2. Fry Consulting Group, Inc. *A Study of Patient's Grievance Mechanisms.* Prepared for the Secretary's Commission on Medical Malpractice. Washington, D.C. U.S. Dept. of Health, Education, and Welfare (undated).
3. Mildred D. Mailick. *Patient Representative Programs in General Short-Term Hospitals and Their Relationship to Social Work.* 1978. (Unpublished dissertation, Columbia University.)
4. Alfred Kahn. *Neighborhood Information Centers.* New York, Columbia University School of Social Work, 1966, pp. 33–35.
5. James Thompson. *Organizations in Action.* New York, McGraw Hill, 1970, pp. 39–40.

Chapter VII

Professionals View Patient Representative Programs

MILDRED D. MAILICK

The previous chapter described the development of patient representative programs in seven hospitals. The most prominent feature was the variability in form and function of each program.

Because patient representative programs lack standardization of their activities, criteria are difficult to establish for evaluating their quality. It is possible, however, to explore the attitudes and opinions of key hospital personnel whose programs most closely have interests in common with those of patient representatives. For this purpose, directors of nursing and social work as well as administrators and patient representatives were interviewed in each of the seven hospitals. They were asked about their attitudes toward and ideas about the patient representative programs as these functioned in their own hospitals, as well as about the idea of patient representation itself.

The Directors of Nursing

There was remarkable uniformity in the responses of directors of nursing to questions about the patient representative programs. They tended to be more favorable to the programs than did either the directors of social work departments or the administrators. While some had reservations about the concept of patient representation in general, they all thought that the programs in their own hospitals were worthwhile. The response of the director of nursing at Barry was typical of those hospitals in which the patient representative programs focused mostly on patient comfort on the inpatient service rather than on grievance and system change.

> Even with nursing complaint and reporting forms, I think there is another legitimate area that the patient representative program fills. On many

occasions, the patient in the hospital is a captive. Patients are threatened by the hospital environment and feel vulnerable . . . A patient may be afraid to complain to a nurse. A patient will say . . . 'she has to take care of me, to give me my pills.' The patient might complain to a patient representative but not a nurse. If the goal is quality patient care, you need patient representatives. Everyone should be alert to problems . . . everyone should communicate, but we still need a patient representative.

In hospitals where the focus of the patient representative program was more connected with monitoring or changing the system, the response of the director of nursing at Farwell reflected the general opinion.

Many people (staff members) are quite capable of resolving an individual patient's problems, but they aren't capable of making impacts on the system. The individual patient's problem may get settled, but the structure doesn't change. Eventually things do change, but with the kind of feedback that a department head gets, it is slow. There is such a time lag before it changes that the individual patient does not feel the problem has been redressed. The patient representative program allows for data collection to take place at the patient care level rather than at the head of department level, as well as to provide immediate response to the patient.

All of the directors of nursing had reservations about the concept of patient representation if it took an adversary stance, and specified that they would be against having that kind of program located in their hospitals. They all felt lucky that the programs had worked out well in their own hospitals although they recognized the possibility that if the present patient representative left that office, an adversary stance could be created by a successor. As the director of nursing at Emerson said:

I know some patient representative programs that are adversary. They antagonize everyone. They 'bomb' in and they don't bother to get all of the facts. Social workers and nurses know that they don't make a judgment until they find out the facts. But they (the patient representatives) barge in. Everyone else is pushed aside.

A number of directors of nursing were thoughtful about the administrative implications of the patient representative programs on their own departments. They emphasized the importance of identifying the position of patient representative as a staff rather than a line position. They were clear that the patient representative should not take over nursing tasks or "fill in" with services that nurses were supposed to perform. They saw the patient representative role as having unique value in that it involves no regular direct service of any kind to the patient, but activates others in the hospital to perform services. Further, representatives can identify gaps in service and bring these to the attention of department heads or administrators.

In line with this, most directors of nursing emphasized the importance of the independence of the patient representative from either nursing or social work departments. They thought that the most appropriate location of the program was within hospital administration, feeling that from that vantage point the patient representative could better monitor other departments.

> I wouldn't want the patient representative to operate out of nursing. Many nurses in supervisory positions get defensive and present a stance that 'my nurse can do no wrong.' What is needed is a check and balance system.

Only one of the directors of nursing was willing to have the program operate from within her department. She felt that if the patient representative had an unambiguous staff function and was not part of the regular line of hierarchy of the nursing department, objectivity and effective monitoring could be maintained. But even she recognized that it would be advantageous for the patient representative not to be a nurse so that loyalties would not become confused.

Not one of the seven directors believed that a nursing background was necessary as preparation for an effective patient representative. They thought that while there might be a slight initial advantage because of the ability of a nurse to master the medical aspects of the problems presented, personal characteristics of general intelligence, tact, stamina, objectivity, and good interpersonal skills were more important. The director of nursing at Emerson thought it was important that the patient representative have some kind of professional knowledge and value base. Until the patient representative group articulated its own code of ethics and provided its own professional training, she believed that, as a protection, the representative should be drawn from some other professional group such as social work or nursing.

In an attempt to assess the priority that directors of nursing placed on the patient representative program in relation to other elements in the hospital system, each was asked to speculate on whether a patient representative program should be set up if there was a scarce resource budget for the hospital. Four out of the seven thought that it would have a low priority in their own way of organizing services in spite of the fact that they approved of the program in their hospitals. They considered the program a frill, not a bare essential. This attitude was exemplified by the director of nursing at Adams.

> From a funding point of view, it has a low priority. Unless we had all else, this would not be our choice. The nursing service are all trained to be patient advocates. Nursing could pick up the program through its own procedures.

The other three directors valued the program highly, and said that they would be quite willing to devote funds to it. Their attitude was that it was worth the investment because it was one method of ensuring the quality of hospital service.

Other methods of quality control were used within their own departments by all of the nursing services in the study. The traditional incident or problem report was the most commonly mentioned mechanism. However, several of the directors recognized that these were limited by the fact that they focused more on individual performance of nurses than on system dysfunction or even gaps in service. Also, they recognized that there could be a considerable time lag between the time an incident occurred and the time the report reached the desk of a director of nursing. Still more time might be taken until enough complaints of a similar nature in any one section of the hospital occurred so that system problems could be identified.

A number of the directors of nursing discussed the nursing audit as an alternative, or, at least, another way of getting data similar to those developed by the patient representative. Two respondents talked about the idea of a process audit which would identify certain patient care problems, develop criteria to measure nursing performance in relation to them, and then systematically evaluate these in one service after another. This method of data collection would rival, the two directors of nursing thought, the best of the data feedback functions of the patient representative programs. Neither of them felt that this would supplant the total purpose of the patient representative program, as they recognized that it monitored more than the nursing function and actively intervened in solving problems for patients.

The Administrators

Of the seven administrators who were interviewed, five considered the patient representative program advantageous to the hospital or to themselves, and two felt it was unnecessary or disadvantageous. In general, in those hospitals where the administrator had been active in starting the program, high value was placed on its functions. The administrator at Emerson was typical of this group. He personally created the position of patient representative, defined its responsibilities, and hired the patient representative. His perception of what a patient representative should or could be went through a series of changes. Although when the program began he conceived of it as being a mechanism of response to patient problems that could not easily be assigned to any of his existing administrative staff, he found, increasingly, that he was relying on the patient representative to study system problems in the hospital. He perceived the patient representative as a personal assistant to him.

> In a way, what she does is a lot of work that you might say ordinarily would be things that I might be getting into, but for lack of time I cannot take care of. This does not diminish her role in responding to patient

complaints. That she pretty much runs. I keep her very busy. She gets through a lot of things I can't get done.

While the administrator at Farwell came to that hospital after the patient representative program had been established, he valued it and had a clear idea of how he wanted to use it. Although he recognized the patient representative as being important in dealing with and resolving patient problems, he found the major rationale for the program in its value to the administration as a feedback mechanism.

If patient care is the primary agenda item of the hospital, then you must have some mechanism for gathering data on what is happening in the institution. I see the patient representative as one dimension of getting information about the care of the patient . . . not the only dimension, but an important one.

The administrator at Caroline valued the patient representative both as a provider of information and some service to the patients and as a monitor of staff attitude toward the patient.

It keeps all staff members on their toes. Some people think that the patient representative must be a headache to me. It really is easier for me to have her. The staff knows that there is a certain level of expectation in responding to patients. They can't just buzz in and buzz out of patients' rooms ignoring their questions. They used to put patients off. Now staff will go into detail in answering questions.

At Davis, the administrator saw the principal value of the patient representative program in the reduction of the number of conflictual incidents between the community and the hospital and the reduction of frustration for individual patients.

The administrators at Adams and Barry had negative valuations of the patient representative program. In each case the administrator felt that the programs were unnecessary and would be abolished if it were not for political considerations. The administrator at Adams was clear about her reasons for opposing the idea.

From a philosophical managerial viewpoint I think it is a really sad commentary that the whole thing [the patient representative program] has ever arisen. Being a manager, my feeling is that a responsible administration shouldn't have to have a patient advocate. I think that a hospital would be much better advised to put its energies into understanding the problem of being more responsive to its patients rather than building another level or system to do that. I think that should be the business of the whole hospital and specifically the business of administration.

At Barry, the administrator had many of the same reservations. He too felt that it was a discredit to a hospital to endorse the need for a patient representative. All but one of the administrators had at least a vague presumption that the presence of a patient representative program in the hospital might cut down on some types of malpractice suits by reducing the frustration level and anger of patients. None of them, however, had any data to prove this, and none saw any way in which the impact of the patient representative program could be assessed. It was only at Emerson that the patient representative was specifically responsible for directly dealing with potential malpractice problems. She was concerned with claims against the hospital by patients who allegedly suffered damage as a result of negligence or malpractice by the hospital staff or attending physicians. The administrator perceived this aspect of the patient representative's activity as most important to the hospital.

Another aspect of the patient representative program that was valued by some of the administrators was the time dimension. Over and over again, it was stressed that physicians, nurses, and social workers all had other professional duties to perform in relation to patients, and that complaints, especially those not central to their own professional tasks, were attended to only when time permitted. The patient representative was seen as someone who would make a patient's complaint a first priority and could follow through without the bureaucratic delays that sometimes occurred, especially when a patient's problem implicated several different systems.

All of the patient representative programs, whatever their other roles or responsibilities, responded at one level or another to patient complaints, and tried to solve problems for individual patients. Except for the program at Guardian, all of the patient representatives claimed to go beyond the complaints of individuals, and either directly or indirectly effect some kind of changes in the system. The administrators in several of the hospitals differed with this perception. For example, while the patient representative at Adams cited examples of change which she was responsible for and which she thought were significant, the administrator thought that the impact of the program on the system was negligible.

> There are things like cleaning up the emergency room. Those kinds of changes occur . . . that is, the level of complaints that eventuate in changes, but not system changes. It is more of a program to get people through the system when something goes wrong and explaining why something went wrong when it did. That is what I think is the problem. They cannot do anything. When you talk about systems, they can't change systems. It has to be on my shoulders.

Similarly, the administrator at Barry saw very little effect on the system of the patient representative program. The patient representative at that hospital gave example after example of ways in which she had moved beyond the request of the patient to try to mediate between systems so as to ensure that patients were more comfortable or better served. The administrator's opinion was that there was no significant change. He made a distinction between system change and process change, although he could not clearly delineate them as two mutually exclusive categories. He suggested that the level of change described by the patient representative related to minor processes rather than to major functions of the hospital.

> The impact of the patient representative program is substantively so minimal and pragmatically such an embarrassment . . . They are always pointing up problems in the system but not solving them. That is not much of a contribution. To my knowledge there have been no changes brought about by the patient representative with basic systemic problems.

The distinction between system and process change was not explicitly made by any of the other administrators. However, the types of changes cited and valued by some of the hospital administrators were probably minor in relation to total hospital functions. For example, at Caroline, one observation of the patient representative was that elderly people tended on hospitalization to suffer from a period of disorientation. They especially seemed to overestimate or underestimate the passage of time. The recommendation of the patient representative was that the hospital equip all of the rooms with clocks. This attention to the comfort of the patient was much valued by the administrator, although he realized that it affected the satisfaction or convenience of the patient more often than the delivery of major services.

Even at Emerson and Davis, where the patient representatives acted as high level administrators, there was recognition of the complexity of the process of systems change and the limitation on the amount of change possible. At Emerson, there were examples of efforts at change of a system nature. One concerned appropriate chart notation. It came to the patient representative's attention that some physicians were using psychiatric terminology in characterizing patients with medical complaints without adequate investigation or documentation. In view of patients' right of access to their charts, there was a general hospital review of notation practices with recommendations for changes all through the hospital.

At Farwell, a number of examples of process change made directly by the patient representative were cited; however, it was clear that the more complex changes were made at higher administrative levels. The contribution of the patient representative was to supply data about patient problems that needed to be evaluated in terms of systems dysfunction.

In sum, the seven administrators had diverse views on the value of patient representative programs and, more importantly, saw them as fulfilling a variety of quite different functions. At one extreme, the patient representative was seen as a personal assistant and, at the other, as an outsider and as an adversary. There was also considerable difference in the estimation of the impact of the program on the hospital. Claims that the patient representative was directly responsible for systemic change came from only one administrator. The rest saw the change as ranging from important to insignificant.

The Directors of Social Work

As in the case of administrators, a wide range of response and valuation of the patient representative program came from directors of social work. There were differences in their views about the concept of patient representation and its rationale, the functions it performed, and its relationship to social work.

All but one of the directors of social work had reservations about what they perceived as the basic idea of patient representation even though some felt that it was working out well in their hospitals. A number of them had questions about the imposition onto an already incredibly complex institution of yet another occupational group that they saw as having no specific function except to take care of the mistakes the system created. This group perceived the patient representative program as a relatively powerless structure, unable to effect any significant change in the system, and responding largely to complaints of patients on a case-by-case basis.

Some social workers suggested that without the possibility of really solving problems on a systems level, the patient representative program had the potential of being harmful or dysfunctional. One called it a "Band-Aid solution." Another suggested

> Anything you throw into the system that helps each individual patient but doesn't affect the system itself only further isolates and alienates. What you create are what I call cynical systems.

Many directors of social work expressed the same idea as the administrators, that is, that the development of a patient representative program in the hospital was somehow a sign of failure, if not at the level of their own department, then of the hospital as a whole. Several of them expressed concern and said that perhaps if the social work department had been more effective or had adopted a more aggressive advocacy stance, the patient representative program might not have gained a foothold in the hospital. Some of the directors saw the patient representative program not as a negative reflection on their own department but as an affront to the hospital administrator.

> How can a hospital administrator say, 'I'm here to serve patients' and then admit that there is a need for patient representatives? Isn't it his job to see to it that everyone in the hospital is showing proper concern for patients? If he finds that he is not doing it well, or that things are getting too complex, then that has to be addressed directly. Don't let the system get

more and more fouled up and throw in a new layer. Straighten out the
system. That's my opinion with patient representatives.

Only one director of social work conceptualized the patient representative program as an aid to the functioning of her department as well
as of the hospital as a whole. She stipulated that she perceived the patient
representative program as being worthwhile only if it performed two
functions: the resolution of individual problems for patients who encountered obstacles in the system, and the development of feedback on patient
care problems occurring in sufficient numbers to require resolution at an
institutional level. She suggested that far from seeing the patient representative program as a sign of failure, she saw it as one mechanism for
ensuring successful functioning. She accepted the fact that a certain
amount of system dysfunction in hospitals is inevitable, and that structures must be developed that would institute correctives for it. Her esti-
mate was that if the hospital as a system worked well 85 to 90 percent of
the time, it was functioning within normal limits, and that as one set of
patient care problems surfaced and were resolved, they would be replaced
by new ones.

> I feel that it is the responsibility of all organizations not to permit more
> and more numbers of the same type of problem to occur. It is an irresponsi-
> ble act. If patient representation is to meet its highest order of responsibil-
> ity, it must feed back data. In the old days we used to say that, therefore,
> the program should ultimately liquidate itself. Now I believe that there
> will always be a need for the program because of the human factor, which
> creates cracks in the system, as well as the institutional factor. Both create
> human problems. So what you get are new surfacing problems which then
> concern you when they come in any volume, and when they do, your
> responsibility is to see that you bring them back for correction.

The directors of social work all saw that there was some relationship
between the functions of their own departments and that of the patient
representatives. There was a range of opinion about what the relationship
was or should be. At one extreme the patient representative and social
work functions were seen as complementary, while at the other, the perception was that they were duplicative and wasteful. Part of this difference
of perception was based on the differences in the patient representative
programs in each hospital as well as the way each of the social work
departments functioned. For example, at Caroline, the patient representative relieved social workers of some unwanted tasks, such as arranging for
the notarizing of wills, the completion of certain forms with which the
patient needed help, and arrangements for transportation. Social workers
were glad to be rid of these activities which they considered peripheral to
their professional role. Similarly, at Adams, the social workers perceived
their work load as being made less burdensome by the introduction of a

patient representative into the waiting area of the emergency room as they no longer were called upon to respond to disruptions there.

In some hospitals, however, the patient representative was seen as a potential threat to the social work department in that the functions performed were sufficiently similar in nature to raise the possibility of conflict and encroachment. One director responded:

> I certainly do think that the patient representative who defines her role as advocacy would be duplicating the social work role. I think that when two different people do the same work under two titles there is waste and trouble.

Another director recounted that while he had not taken it seriously, one administrator in his hospital had proposed that the social work department could be replaced by a combination of lawyers and patient representatives who would force the doctors and nurses into being more responsive to patients.

Yet other social work directors saw the potential of the patient representative program for providing a valuable service that augmented the social work function. At Farwell, the patient representative program was seen as one of the mechanisms for the delivery of social work services.

> The philosophy on which we established the patient representative function out of the social work department is that social work is related to a problem-solving approach not only in relation to the person needing health care, but to the system as well. When the system breaks down in terms of offering the individual appropriate care, that is a social work service problem. I am not talking about a major breakdown in the total hospital that might occur if, for example, the entire x-ray department isn't working. That is an administrative problem. I am saying that when an individual (patient) has met an impediment in the system, it has a natural place in social work.

A number of directors dealt with the idea that perhaps the patient representative could perform a unique function by virtue of being outside the regular hierarchy of the social work department. They thought that the line social workers might become overly identified with the staff of the unit or service area to which they were assigned, and therefore be less sensitive to needs of patients especially when these conflicted with staff or system needs, or which, when pursued too vigorously by social workers, jeopardized work relationships.

One social work director expressed her concern:

> I think sometimes the worker tends to be coopted by the system and may not always have either the correct identification or, even more importantly, the correct power base to be a true advocate. For that reason, I think it is generally better to have advocates outside of a normal departmental system.

At Caroline, the lack of identification of the patient representative with the staff of the service area or unit was emphasized as a negative. The thought was that the patient representative might overreact on behalf of the patient.

> Social workers don't get so over-identified with the patient. We don't always think the patient is right. We also have more ongoing relationships with a group of doctors and other staff members, and can't risk in the same way that volunteers [patient representatives] do. We are more careful. I think sometimes we raise problems, but we try to be more tactful. We don't just criticize. The patient representative just comes to a quick conclusion, but the social worker is more analytical in her assessment of the problem.

Most social work directors were ambivalent about whether, if given the opportunity, they would want to have the patient representative program lodged within the social work department. This seemed to be connected with their views of their own departments and their views of the function of social work. The director at Davis, a public hospital which had just undergone severe budget cuts and constriction of the size of the staff of the social work department, described her current view of social work in her hospital.

> The essential service given in this building is medical treatment. Anything that is not absolutely essential to that main function is being eliminated. When you get down to that point, they can do without social service except around discharge planning. We are needed to get people out of the hospital so others can come in.

Since she saw the necessity of focusing the activity of her department very narrowly, and since she felt relatively powerless in the hospital decision-making process, she thought that the patient representative function would not be well served within her department.

The director of social work at Guardian felt that advocacy for patients was definitely a core responsibility of social work, and therefore she saw the patient representative function as part of her domain. While she indicated that in principle she would want to place the patient representative program within her department, in practice she would not fight for it. This was because the program at her hospital was weak, and her own position in the bureaucracy would not lead her to fight for a failing program.

Similar attitudes were held by the directors of social work at Emerson and Adams. At Emerson, the director was unsure about the advisability of placing the patient representative program within her domain.

> Off the top of my head I would say no. It is not anything I would be against if the suggestion came from outside of the department, but it is not anything I would go out and seek.

At Adams, the director saw both advantages and disadvantages to the idea. Conceptually, she saw the role of social work as including advocacy functions. Outside of the emergency room, in which the patient representative program based its activities, the social work department provided a variety of advocacy services. But the director was not sure that she would want the patient representative program within her department. Her reasoning was very much like that of the director of social work at Guardian. Since the program was initiated from outside the hospital and was poorly valued by the administration, the social work department was not eager to "own" it.

At Caroline as well as at Emerson the directors of social work were satisfied to have the patient representative program remain outside the social work department because of the excellent relationships with the incumbent patient representative. However, they were quick to state that they might change their opinions if the current patient representative were to be replaced.

At Farwell, the patient representative program was already lodged in the social work department. The director saw the "patient to system breakdown" as just as important a point of intervention for social work as helping the patient cope with the problems created by the illness. Although she expected that all of the line social workers had the responsibility of regularly assessing their practice for system problems, she valued the overall system view of the patient representative and her capacity to gather data from across service boundaries. Organizationally, the director thought that the patient representative was best situated outside of the regular line hierarchy of the social work department, reporting directly to her. Data about patient care problems of the entire outpatient service were then communicated at the appropriate level to the various services or turned over to administration for problem resolution.

The director of social work at Farwell saw the patient representative as only one aspect of the larger effort at controlling the quality of service in the department. She saw it as being complementary to two other quality assurance programs that were built into the Medicaid and Medicare regulations: peer review and service audits. Both of these assessment techniques, however, deal with closed cases and retrospective evaluation; the patient representative program offered an after-the-fact corrective dealing with more immediate problems and thus added another dimension.

Some of the social work directors expressed doubts about the impact of the program on the hospital system and on their own department. The director at Barry recognized that systemic change was complex and difficult to accomplish. He did not think that the patient representative program as it was constituted in his hospital was capable of managing it.

> I don't see them [the patient representatives] making any kind of institutional change. I don't think that social work can make any change acting alone. We can if the hospital is interested in it and if others are involved.

Even at Farwell, where the patient representative was part of the social work department, the director saw limitations in the capacity of the program to deal with highly complex issues. She also observed that the patient representative responded only to those problems about which the patient complained. This gave a very selective view of the problems in the hospital. Another potential issue she raised was that when it became known in the system that the patient representative could handle a certain type problem, more and more of the same kinds of complaints would be directed to her. The danger is that the patient representative would develop a series of institutionalized problem-solving tasks rather than push the system toward direct resolution of the problems.

Thus, the directors of social work responded to a variety of issues about patient representation with thoughtfulness and concern. While two out of the seven directors of the programs would have been ready to abolish the programs outright if they could, the rest had a range of opinions about the potential of the programs. Several anticipated that there might be trouble if the two functions became more antagonistic as a result of changes in the staffing of the patient representative program.

The Patient Representatives

All of the patient representatives were highly enthusiastic about their jobs and eager to describe what they did. They were aware of the existence of different types of patient representative programs in other hospitals, but made few comparative statements between their own and other programs. In most cases their estimation of the positive contribution of their programs to the functioning of the hospitals was very high. While some thought that their impact was direct and a consequence of their own actions, others felt that their main effect was catalytic and that their influence was largely indirect. At Davis, the patient representative felt that she was effective as a result of direct action.

> I can call the doctors and read them the riot act. They don't like it, but that's tough. They are afraid of me because I am an associate director of the hospital. I don't answer to anybody but the director. Any problem I see that needs change on an administrative level, I work out. I decide on the changes I see that need to be made, and I present it to the executive director's meeting. Usually I have done my homework well, and I don't have any fight out of them.

At Emerson, the patient representative also saw her program as having a direct impact, but her description of the way she went about her work was different from that described by the patient representative at Davis.

My power is only because people are willing to deal with me and work with me. In 99.9 percent of the situations, it is my informal power that works. If I want to make a change, first I have to convince the people it is going to affect that it is a needed one. Then they have to work with me to set up a system they can live with. Then I have to get administration to approve it. All I am doing is getting everybody together. I am not really coming out with a fiat saying that this is going to be it.

The patient representative at Caroline thought that she had considerable impact, but recognized that it was largely indirect in nature.

The patient representative sort of plants the seed, then nursing will discuss it or the medical board will discuss it. We sort of start things going. It is very hard to say that we have radically changed anything, but what we have caused to happen is that everybody seems to care . . . they are more aware of patient needs.

At Adams, the patient representative was realistic about the limits of her power:

This hospital is very polite on the surface. There are times when issues need to be faced. But sometimes you can get more by not forcing. When we engage in providing information to patients, and that is our major role, it is very well accepted by everybody, but when an attempt is made to go beyond that, questions are raised. If we keep to the job of allaying a patient's anxiety, it is OK, but if I see something amiss with the doctors, my power is such that I can't get into that very easily.

The patient representative at Farwell felt that while she accomplished much by direct action, there were limits beyond which she could not go.

There are limits to how much I can push. But they are usually budgetary limits. I have not had that much conflict with any administrator. That doesn't mean I have gotten everything done that I have asked for. On the important things, I have gotten some work done. Nothing that I have wanted to push has been just ignored. If I can't get it done now, then I at least know that it is being worked on. Some things need to be worked on for a long time.

The patient representatives all felt that they made a unique contribution to the hospital by functioning in a mediating role, making judgments about when the complaints of the patient were justified and when the hospital staff was right. They wrestled with the problem of dual identification with the hospital and the patient.

At Emerson, the patient representative felt that the issue was overemphasized.

> My concern is about what is basically right. Many times when I get
> involved in something, people will say, 'Oh, you are obviously only for the
> hospital,' or 'Oh, you are only for the patient.' I have trouble sorting that
> out because I don't see it as one or the other. If you can help the hospital
> do a better job, isn't that better for the patient? I am here to protect both,
> because if you only protect one, it is not sufficient. They affect each other.

The patient representative at Davis also saw herself as a mediator, but
her stance was much more aggressive in promoting what she thought was
the patient's position.

> When my boss wants me to keep something quiet that I think is wrong,
> I am going to scream to high heaven. Why else has he got me here? If he
> fires me, I am going to the newspapers and make a wave like he never saw,
> and he knows it. I think sometimes he is sorry that he put me in this job.
> But this is a big hospital and people are getting walked all over every day.
> If I am not here to scream and holler then there is no reason to have me
> here.

At Caroline, the patient representative was more unassuming in her
perception of her mediating role.

> Perhaps we are not the advocate in the true sense, because our relationship
> here is very dual. We love the patients and we love the hospital. We sort
> of watch out for both sides.

The patient representative at Farwell was quite clear about her own
personal stance:

> As far as I am concerned, I am here for the patient. Everything I do is
> for the patient. Now that doesn't mean that there aren't times when I can't
> say, 'This patient is not right,' or even, judgmentally, 'The patient really
> shouldn't get something he wants.' But my philosophy is that all my
> dealings with the patient or with trying to change the system are focused
> on what is going to be easier or fairer for the patient.

A number of patient representatives drew attention to their role in
relation to the *Patient's Bill of Rights.* The patient representative at Emerson expressed the position of all of those interviewed:

> I don't believe the *Patient's Bill of Rights* [can be implemented]. It is a
> worthless piece of paper. It is mandated in the State of New York as part
> of the health code. But how do you enforce what they put in there—that
> every patient is entitled to respect? We have 5,000 employees. I can't
> guarantee that 24 hours a day every single one of the employees is going
> to be respectful and courteous. But there are some things that do have a
> legal basis: informed consent, confidentiality of the patient's record and

diagnosis, and the right to privacy. Those are legal doctrines and there I have concern—that the patient have his legal rights honored.

The patient representatives had much to say about what they thought about the educational and personal qualifications of the patient representative, issues of professionalization, and the role of volunteers. The group was fairly unanimous in the idea that the patient representative did not have to be either a nurse or social worker or have any specific professional training at all. The question was whether completion of a bachelor's degree should be the minimal educational requirement. The patient representative at Farwell, who had a B.A., suggested that this was a source of controversy whenever the patient representatives got together at a national convention, and that there were strong feelings about it. Her point of view was:

> I think that if you are really going to do a good job you have to deal on an equal basis with administrators and top people in the hospital, and you have to be comfortable doing it. If the B.A. . . . helps, then I think it is necessary. I think that there are some people who do not have the B.A. who can do the job, but basically if you have a large hospital and a complex hierarchy, you need to have the qualifications of whomever else you are going to deal with.

The patient representative at Emerson was more specific about what the educational content should be:

> There are a lot of things that I think a patient representative needs. Probably it has to be at the master's degree level, but maybe it could be at a four-year college level. I think you need a psychology background, a knowledge of sociology, anatomy and physiology, the health care delivery system, and the legislative things that affect health care. You should understand reimbursement and what it means to patient care.

Most of the other patient representatives felt that no special educational background was important. One had a strong antiprofessional bias, and expressed the feeling that nurses and social workers were really unsuited for patient representation. She felt that their education and professional identification might blind them to certain problems and generally remove them from the patient. She saw advantages in her own lay background and her lack of a college education. She thought her minority status was an additional asset.

All of the patient representatives thought that personal attributes were more important than formal education. They valued intelligence, tact, communication skills, political expertise, compassion, the capacity to deal with anger, and, when necessary, to be aggressive and to fight. These were characteristics that they felt patient representatives brought to the job. In addition, they had to know the resources and operations of each part of the hospital in great detail.

There was diversity of opinion about the issue of whether patient representation could be considered as a profession. The two patient representatives who most favored a college degree as a minimum requirement for entry into the job also identified themselves as part of a profession. Both were active in the founding of the Society of Patient Representatives. One served as the first president of the national organization and the other was president at the time of the study. While they were aware of the diversity of types of programs and people employed as patient representatives, they looked forward to a process in which the least qualified of the group would be replaced gradually by college educated, career-minded individuals.

Another position was taken by the patient representative at Davis who was antiprofessional in her stance. She saw the job of patient representative as a stepping-stone, a transitional stage in which no one should remain over a long period of time. She was, in addition, disappointed in the national organization, which she felt was interested in promoting the interests of patient representatives rather than the interests of patients.

Three of the other patient representatives interviewed belonged to the national organization, but were not interested or active in it. They tended to identify themselves more with the hospital than with the occupational grouping. They saw their employment more as a job than a profession and derived their occupational self-esteem more from their relationships to colleagues in the hospital than to other patient representatives.

Except for the patient representative program at Guardian, all of the programs had used the services of the volunteers at one time or another, and in a variety of capacities. In three of the programs, volunteers were central to the operation of the service. At Adams, the bulk of the service was delivered by volunteers. This required constant recruitment and training because of the high rate of turnover among the volunteer group. In addition there were many problems in recruiting lower socioeconomic group volunteers as required by the grant agreement, as few offered their services. The utilization of the services of those who were recruited was accompanied by difficulties. While the lower socioeconomic class volunteers related quite well to patients in the emergency room, the hospital staff was less accepting of them than of middle class volunteers and some friction developed. The patient representative who directed the program felt that in spite of these problems, she valued the volunteer group highly, and thought they added a special quality to her program.

Volunteers at Caroline were also highly valued by the patient representative. The social status of this group was important as they all had had a long relationship and commitment to service to the hospital, and many of them were either board members or had social connections with them.

The volunteer patient representatives were offered a three-month course of training by the patient representative program, during which they were introduced to the functions and activities of every department of the hospital. In contrast to Adams, there had been almost no turnover in the volunteer group, and so the long training period was worthwhile.

At Barry, where the program was originally started by volunteers, the relationship between the paid patient representative and the volunteers was quite complicated. Since the volunteers provided funding for the program, they were, in effect, the employers of the patient representative but, at the same time, they were supervised by her.

Three other programs placed volunteers in ancillary positions, but they had less influence on the nature of the program. At Farwell, volunteers provided a good part of the information and referral services, and at Emerson they did casefinding. The patient representative at Emerson commented:

> My response to the question of the use of volunteers as patient representatives is that first, you must define the purpose of the patient representative program. If it is involved in providing for the personal comfort of the patient, then volunteers can do very well, but not when it comes to problem solving. Volunteers can listen to patients and engage in conversation with them. They can help a patient remove himself from the sick atmosphere for a period of time. Perhaps the patient needs some laundry sent out, something mailed, the traditional personal services that volunteers have always given. If that is how you define the patient representative function then you can use volunteers. It seems wasteful of money to pay someone to do what volunteers have done fantastically well for years. But if you define the patient representative as a mechanism for the patient to have a grievance resolved, I don't want a volunteer involved. They are here one day a week if you are lucky, and how do you train them? They have no right to a patient's chart and why should the doctor talk to them?

Thus, a wide range of opinion was expressed by the patient representative group on all issues. To a large extent, they valued the form of program in their own hospitals, accepted its rationale, and reflected ideas and attitudes that were consonant with their own experiences. They were thoughtful about such issues as the impact of their programs on the hospitals, troubled by the conflict of dual identification, and concerned about issues of professionalization.

Chapter VIII

The Society of Patient Representatives

RUTH RAVICH

Patient representatives as an occupational group emerged in the late 1960's during the period of rapid technological change and increasing division of labor in the medical field. It is one of more than 50 occupational groups now employed in health care institutions. Many of these groups require a high degree of expertise in a narrow area of specialization, perfusionists, x-ray technicians, and genetic counselors, for example. Patient representation is unique, however, in that its major raison d'être is to counter the negative effects and to facilitate the benefits of increased technology. Its practitioners are not specialists, but generalists trained to look at health care settings from the patients' point of view.

The patient representative group also differs from the technical specialty groups in that much of its initial support came from a general movement toward human rights rather than from a need perceived by the health care professions. The United Hospital Fund of New York, the Greater New York Hospital Association, and the American Hospital Association (AHA), recognized the value of patient representatives in the delivery of health care in the early 1970's. Their interest and support had a powerful influence on the course of development and the rapid growth of the field.

The Association of Patient Service Representatives

In August 1969, the Training Research and Special Studies Division of the United Hospital Fund of New York invited a patient representative from three hospitals—The Mount Sinai Hospital and Long Island Jewish Hospital in New York, and Temple University Hospital in Philadelphia, Pennsylvania—to assist in exploring the possibilities of extending patient representative services to more hospitals. A seminar was sponsored by the

United Hospital Fund and the Greater New York Hospital Association and planned by the three patient representatives who had been working in complete isolation from each other unaware of common activities and problems. They decided to meet after the seminar to continue the exchange of ideas and working methods.

The seminar, or workshop, held in New York in April 1970, for hospital directors, department heads, patient representatives, and patient relations managers addressed such issues as the role of the patient representative, resources needed for an effective program, placement within the hospital organizational structure, separation from other hospital functions, relationships to other departments and the importance of administrative commitment. Because of the enthusiastic evaluations, additional workshops were planned.

A second workshop, held in New York City in October 1970, examined the basic philosophies underlying the appointment of patient representatives, the involvement of administration, approaches to individual patient problems, compilation of statistics, and use of these data to help administration move toward needed change. The exchange of ideas was so helpful to many of those attending that a committee was selected to form an association. At a meeting held in December 1970, the committee decided that the organization would be called the Association of Patient Service Representatives. Committee members agreed to contact hospitals in the Northeast to obtain information on existing programs, and to offer membership to representatives in them.

A third workshop, "Looking at the Hospital from the Patient's Point of View," was held in Philadelphia in the spring of 1971. The 140 people attending included hospital administrators, patient representatives, hospital public relations officers, and representatives of AHA, the press, and the public. Fifty-five health care institutions in nine states were represented. An executive committee was chosen to apply for a charter and to write by-laws. The executive committee soon realized that resources for locating and contacting other patient representatives throughout the country and for mounting meetings and workshops were not available within the association. Because of this limitation, the group decided to petition for establishment as an affiliated society of the AHA.

The statement of philosophy and goals that the Association of Patient Service Representatives presented to the AHA clearly indicated a dedication to maintaining the dignity and integrity of patients. A patient representative was described as an individual in the organization responsible for assuring each patient the best and most courteous care the institution was capable of providing. Patient needs were to be expeditiously met in an individualized manner. Patient representatives were to identify and document problem areas in the provision of services so that the care and treatment of patients could be continuously reevaluated by administrative and medical staff. In this way, patient representatives would serve as catalysts, stimulating appropriate action that would result in improved patient care. Patient representatives were conceived of as representing both patients and the medical facility, and were to reconcile these elements to the ultimate satisfaction of patients.

Two goals for the new organization were proposed. The first was to make administrators of health care facilities and consumers of health care cognizant of the value of patient service representation to patients and to the institution, and to assist in the development of programs. The second was to organize training institutes to consider modalities for: a) coping with individual patient and procedural problems, b) relating to different levels of medical and administrative management, c) establishing effective reportorial mechanisms, and d) working with community groups and consumer advocates to improve hospital and ambulatory care for all consumers.

Development of the Society

On September 23, 1971, members of the AHA staff met with the executive committee of the Association of Patient Service Representatives to discuss affiliation. A recommendation made to the AHA Board was approved, and the patient representatives group became the thirteenth affiliated AHA member society. Its aim, to promote the work of patient representatives, reflected the AHA's concern for helping its member institutions bring greater understanding of hospitals to consumers. It was also anticipated that the society would act as a conduit to bring consumer concerns and needs to the attention of the health care industry.

The AHA affiliation provided financial and staff support, and advanced the acceptance of the new occupation by publicizing the role of the patient representative to AHA member hospitals. Acceptance under the umbrella of the AHA did much to enhance the status of the occupation, as the organization of patients representatives joined AHA affiliates whose membership was restricted to management personnel and professionals: hospital nursing service administrators, purchasing management, social service directors and personnel administration. Some patient representatives believed that this early acceptance of the infant association by the AHA was a strategy for control of a group that otherwise might become part of a strong consumer movement acting in an adversary role toward institutions represented by the AHA. Another concern was a requirement that Society members be employed by AHA member institutions. This regulation excluded many active patient advocates who were employed by nonmember institutions, including some municipal hospitals and in community advocacy programs, groups which could be expected to make valuable contributions to the field.

In November 1971, a questionnaire was sent by the AHA to administrators of member hospitals requesting information about existing patient representative programs and offering membership to patient representatives employed by them. An advisory panel met in January 1972 to adopt a name, develop bylaws, prepare a statement of objectives and present a slate of candidates for election to the first board of directors of the group. A mail ballot was sent to the 122 patient representatives who had accepted membership.

Adopting a Name

The Association of Patient Service Representatives, when it organized in 1971, elected to include "service" in its title because a patient representative links a patient to hospital services, and also represents patients in the system. In affiliating with the AHA, the advisory panel eliminated the word "service," and the association became the Society of Patient Representatives. Members, however, have not yet accepted a common title, and function under a variety of titles. At the second annual meeting in 1973, 76 of the 106 registrants used titles that indicated their function in dealing with patients' concerns and problems or with the amenities of patient care; 22 were called patient representatives; 16 patient service representatives or coordinators; 16 had appointments in patient relations departments; 11 were listed as ombudsmen or advocates; 3 were patient counselors; and 2 listed themselves as hostesses. Other related titles were patient affairs office, patient administration, and patient communications.

In 1978, 189 Society members participated in the annual meeting and workshop. In this group, 18 different titles indicating direct patient assignments were listed. One hundred and six or 57 percent of this group were listed as patient representatives, indicating a shift toward acceptance of this title.

In some institutions the title, patient representative, is used by members of finance and billing departments, not by a staff member acting on a patient's behalf. In an attempt at clarification, this point was brought to a joint committee of the AHA and the Hospital Financial Management Association (HFMA) in 1976. One recommendation to the Joint Committee was that the word "financial" or "fiscal" be included in the title of persons concerned with matters of financial management. The recommendation was not accepted by the HFMA, and the matter was referred back to AHA staff for further consideration. The use of the same title by staff members with diverse functions is of continuing concern to the Society of Patient Representatives as it causes considerable confusion for many patients. However, since the AHA has not been able to resolve the issue, members have been asked to address the problem in their individual hospitals.

Bylaws

The bylaws drawn by the Advisory Panel were approved at the first meeting of the society held in Chicago in October 1972.

The Society's objectives are:

To promote the improvement and extension of adequate health services to all persons and to advance the development of effective patient representative programs in health care institutions by:

a. conducting educational programs and activities to strengthen and develop patient representative programs,

b. providing a medium for the interchange of ideas and information among members, and,

c. disseminating information on patient representative programs to health care institutions and agencies.

The concern about membership restricted to employees of AHA member institutions was resolved by a clause in the bylaws of the new society that opened up to 49 percent of the membership in local chapters to patient advocates affiliated with nonmember hospitals. In 1975, the AHA opened its personal membership to all interested parties with or without affiliations in associated hospitals and to community representatives without hospital appointments. Few, if any, who are not affiliated with health care institutions have availed themselves of this membership opportunity. *If* the founders were correct in their assumption that individuals functioning as patient advocates outside of health care institutions would lend vitality and would be an asset to the society, this potential source of support is as yet untapped.

Membership

At the invitation of the AHA, 122 members had joined the Society before the first meeting. Many states were represented, and area representatives were appointed in seven of the nine AHA regional districts. Their role was to answer inquiries about patient representation and provide information to hospital administrators considering programs. Before 1973 ended, membership had more than doubled with 281 members from 42 states, including Hawaii, as well as the District of Columbia, the Canal

Zone, and Canada. By 1974, working guidelines developed by the Society were being used as far afield as Colombia, South America. In 1974 only 45 new members joined the Society, but there has been a steady gain of approximately 100 new members a year since then. In October 1978, at the 7th Annual Meeting, membership stood at 708, representing 48 states, Canada, and Washington, D.C. In the spring of 1979, there were 750 members on the roster. Nine chapters had formally affiliated; the first was New York/New Jersey in 1974, followed by Illinois/Indiana/Kentucky, Wisconsin, Colorado, Sunshine (Florida), Kansas/Missouri, Potomac (Washington, D.C.), Pennsylvania, and Oregon.

Delineating the Role

During the first year, four major patient representative functions were identified: "*Outreach*—to seek out those individuals who need services, link the individuals to services, link the services within the institution, and help facilitate communication among components of the system; *Advocate*—to identify the obstacles to service, investigate the source of difficulty, determine an appropriate course of action, and document and communicate findings to administration or that service which can effect change; *Educator-Mobilizer*—to participate in activities both within the institution and in the community which will personalize and humanize delivery of services to patients; *Data Manager*—to provide appropriate hospital departments with specific information relating to impediments to the delivery of services."

The tasks outlined were: interviewing individuals in need of service, providing information about services and interpreting the institution's policy and procedures; documenting and reporting results of patient interviews, including satisfaction with and/or obstacles to delivery of service; following through by resolving problems directly and making referrals, making recommendations for change in existing policies and procedures to appropriate departments or services; following up by checking with the department or service involved as to its decision and implementation of that decision; interpreting the patient representative role to patients, staff, and community.

While the Society has defined basic functions of representatives, there is still considerable role variation among its members. Each hospital determines the scope of its program and defines the responsibilities to fit its own (the hospital's) needs. A manual published by the Society states:

"In many instances a successful approach to achieving acceptance of a patient representative program is to begin with a program focusing on personal needs of patients. Once both the concept and the person responsible for carrying out the program are accepted, hospital staff itself often provides the impetus for further development and expansion of the patient representative program."[1]

Reflected in this statement is the perception that determination of occupational boundaries involves a process of negotiation within each institution. Some of the factors that influence this process are the title used, administrative authority granted for the performance of certain functions, and the relationships of the representatives with other staff. Most new patient representatives are selected from within the organization. A need for negotiation is seen in relationships between patient representatives, social workers, nurses, and middle-level administrators. Many of them criticize patient representatives for invading their territory and usurping some of their functions. Social workers in particular comment that the roles of patient advocate and change agent are ones they should be performing.

In order to better define the patient representative role vis-a-vis that of social workers, a statement was issued jointly by the AHA's societies of Patient Representatives and Hospital Social Work Directors. The guidelines suggest that social workers' responsibilities are "to help patients and their families with social, environmental and emotional problems associated with their illness; to help them in using prescribed medical care; to provide aftercare planning; and to make referrals to community agencies . . .". Patient representatives' responsibilities are "to assist patients, their families and hospital staff members to recognize and remove institutional obstacles to providing high quality health care."[2] A simple rule of thumb is that if patients "can't cope with the system," they should be handled by patient representatives. If patients "can't cope," they should be referred to social workers.

Qualifications:

In 1973, the Society's Committee on Career Definition, appointed at the first meeting of the Society, submitted its recommendation on qualifications for patient representatives, which were approved by the members. They recommended that the director of a department have a bachelor's degree and at least four years of paid professional experience in the field of human services or an equivalent combination of people-oriented experience and training. The assistant director should have a bachelor's degree and at least two years of paid professional experience in the field of human services, or an equivalent combination of people-oriented experience and training. Recommendations for entry level positions of patient representative were: a bachelor's degree with relevant experience, including paid professional work, extracurricular activities or volunteer work;graduation from a school of nursing and additional experience; an associate of arts degree and two years paid experience, or a high school diploma and at least four years of appropriate experience. Entry level patient representatives were expected to enhance skills through such relevant continuing education courses as psychology, sociology, and medical terminology.

These recommendations became an issue at the annual meeting in San Francisco in 1974 in the first open clash of opinions faced by the Society when an organized subgroup took the floor to argue against academic qualifications for patient representatives. The group stated that academic preparation might disqualify a candidate as high educational achievement would create a large gap between advocates and those most needing their help (the poor and the disadvantaged). The issue was referred back to committee. During the height of the debate one patient representative who held a M.D. degree argued that education per se did not obviate the ability to relate to and help those with less education. Few of the central city advocacy programs manned by indigenous personnel, with little formal education, have survived. The reason for the demise of many of these programs was a shift in allocation of OEO funds by which they were supported. There has been no evaluation as to whether academic preparation or the lack of it contributed to this change. To the present, no alternative educational recommendations have been formulated. As an increasing number of patient representatives assume the responsibility of department head, more of these appointees have college and postgraduate training.

In 1973, responses to a questionnaire sent to Society members indicated that 24 percent had bachelor's or postgraduate degrees. In 1976 this figure was 44 percent: 34 percent bachelor's and 10 percent master's degrees.

In the absence of a requirement for educational qualifications, the personal capacities of the patient representative takes on greater importance. The committee on career definition suggested that maturity, tact, judgment, flexibility, sensitivity, empathy, tenacity, communication skills, sense of humor, and ability to cope with stress were the qualities that were most helpful in performance of the job.

In addition to the tasks of patient representatives described above, the director of a department would be expected to:

—Plan, organize, direct and evaluate the program.

—Orient and train patient representatives.

—Supervise staff and volunteers assigned to the department.

—Establish and maintain effective working relationships with patients, other staff members, and the community.

—Maintain documentation for recommending changes in hospital policy and procedures.

—Participate in inservice education.

The patient representative group has thus suggested qualifications for members, but it is the employing institution that makes decisions about its own needs. Membership is granted according to title and job description to those whose major role in the health care institution is to represent patients. The Society of Patient Representatives has not attempted to restrict entrance into the group according to educational or other qualifications.

One of the questions dealt with from the inception of the organization was the need for a systematic body of knowledge or theory drawn up by the practitioner in making operational decisions. This implies a period of academic training as preparation for the role. Whether the Society should determine necessary content and how to make the information available in an organized manner, perhaps through an academic curriculum, was discussed at a meeting of the board of directors in October 1973. It was pointed out that in seeking to stabilize the knowledge base of the organization, standards should not exclude persons who could perform effectively. A committee on education was appointed to look into the benefits and problems associated with encouraging or sponsoring a formal academic curriculum.

Over succeeding years, several colleges and universities have approached the Society for collaboration in such programs. In 1978 the board voted to continue to offer educational workshops and seminars at semiannual meetings and to encourage local chapters to do likewise, but not to participate in any formal educational curriculum being offered by educational institutions.

Continuing Education Activities

In lieu of support for formal academic courses, the Society has taken an alternate step of upgrading the knowledge and skills of its members by offering educational programs.

A series of workshops are held at each annual meeting and are supplemented by yearly regional programs. The topics chosen for these workshops mirror the concerns of a group growing in sophistication and sense of its own purpose. During the first few years focus was placed on establishing patient representative programs and accomplishing tasks. Seminars included: organizing a patient representative program, setting goals and defining roles, communication skills, interdisciplinary interaction, influencing staff attitudes, and establishing relations with the community. As programs developed, it was apparent that only a small number of the institution's patient population who needed or would benefit from assistance by a patient representative would be reached. While these might be served effectively without record-keeping, system change that would make the institution more responsive to all patients could not be achieved without documentation. Methods for recording and reporting were presented in workshops on: verbal and written communication, documentation and statistical reports, and the role of the change agent.

Educational sessions after the first few years reflect the expanding roles of the membership. In 1975 optional sessions were offered to new practitioners. Experienced members began to deal with such subjects as power theory and institutional changes; trends in health care; child abuse, rape and abortion; discharge planning; legal aspects of the patient representative's responsibility; legislation relevant to hospitals; patient's rights; and the role of the volunteer in patient representative programs. Special interest sessions offered discussions on pastoral care, ethical issues, and cultural variations in the acceptance of health care.

As many of the patient representative departments became integral components of the institutions' administrative structure, seminars began to deal with management skills and styles, long-range planning and establishing goals, budgeting, and special funding. Evaluating the effectiveness of programs, cost benefit, and cost containment, were added subjects.

By providing workshops on methods of evaluation, the Society expects to encourage the membership to undertake evaluative studies. The first of these, a workshop on time studies, was offered at the 1978 annual meeting. A committee to develop guidelines and provide assistance for evaluative studies has been appointed. Although to date no evaluative studies have been reported, in the perception of many practitioners and hospital administrators patient representative departments reduce hospital costs by cutting across departmental lines to solve problems quickly and effectively, providing a central point for grievances to be aired, eliminating the need for patients to discuss their concerns with many different staff members.

Patient representatives have been active in the implementation of patients' rights in their hospitals since 1973, and many meetings and workshops have been offered on drafting and implementing of the *Patients' Bill of Rights* for individual hospitals and on methods for informing patients of their rights and establishing grievance procedures for those who feel there has been infringement. The Society responded to the legal implications of patient advocacy by offering a series of workshops including patients' rights and patient grievance mechanisms and law for the layman. Legislation mandating dissemination of patients' rights information and patients' grievance mechanisms was passed by the state of Colorado in 1973 and Minnesota in 1976, and is projected in several other state legislatures. By 1976 this legislation was also being discussed in the Congress. In May of 1977, a member of the United States Congress officially informed the Society that he was interested in proposing legislation mandating patient representatives in health care institutions. This was opposed by the Society's Board of Directors because of its mandatory nature. In the board's view, a patient representative program, to be effective, must have the real support of the hospital board and administration, and the trust, support, and cooperation of staff. It was felt that mandating such programs often results in tokenism rather than truly effective operational programs and results in rigidity and inflexibility in a program whose effectiveness is the direct result of its ability to adapt and to be flexible. Mandating could also result in patient representatives being viewed by other staff members as policemen or adversaries rather than as members of the health care team. Patients also may be intimidated by such formal "legal" mechanisms, further jeopardizing the effectiveness of patient representatives.

Despite these reasons for opposing legislation, the board agreed that the Society should be prepared to offer positive suggestions to those who insisted on pursuing mandated programs. A committee, composed of members from states where legislation already affected patient representatives in hospitals and other health care institutions and from states where such legislation was pending, was appointed to address the issue. In addition, the Society developed guidelines for patient representatives in a model patient grievance system.[3] The Report of the American Bar Association Commission on Medical Liability contains a chapter on patients' rights and responsibilities in which it is recommended that hospitals strongly consider providing a mechanism such as patient representative for the resolution of patient problems and complaints and the protection of patients' rights.

The role of the patient representative in hospital risk management programs is another topic that has come to the fore as members assume increasingly responsible roles in this area. The St. Paul Fire and Marine Insurance Company recommended that patient representative be included in hospitals' risk management programs. The New Jersey Board of Insurance Underwriters has ordered a 2 percent premium surcharge to those insured hospitals that do not comply with a requirement that each patient, on admission, be advised on how to report complaints, that each patient's complaints be reviewed by a central source, acted upon, and a record kept of the followup. Workshop sessions at the meetings in 1977–1978 offered a variety of models to enable each participant to choose one most appropriate to his/her institution and discuss the issues with others working in similar settings.

Use of Volunteers:

The use of volunteers in patient representative departments is of continued concern in this new health care occupation. Some hospitals use volunteers as an adjunct to the program and some have an all-volunteer department. Over the years many programs developed by volunteers have found it essential to employ at least one full-time paid staff person to maintain continuity. On one hand, the use of volunteers is encouraged even in well-staffed departments as the extra personnel can add to the number of contacts with patients. Volunteers can be effective in informing patients about hospital facilities and regulations, and can assist with patients who need more attention and support than other staff are able to provide. They can be very effective in humanizing and individualizing the hospital experience. Volunteers can provide these services within budget constraints, but it is felt that the extensive use of volunteers may dilute effectiveness and limit program development. The change agent role in particular often requires delicate maneuvering by a staff person who is an integral member of the health care team. The Society, in conjunction with the AHA Society of Directors of Volunteer Services, has developed guidelines for use of volunteers in patient representative programs, which define the value of the volunteer in certain aspects of the patient representative role and suggests limitations on involvement in others.[4]

The Role of the Society in the Larger Health Care Community

The Society's role extends beyond its own membership in its efforts to advance the number and effectiveness of patient representative programs. Members of the Society have served on important national and AHA committees: The Secretary's (HEW) Commission on Medical Malpractice; the Joint Committee of the American Psychiatric Association and the American Hospital Association dealing with psychosocial needs of hospitalized patients; the Committee on Health Care for the Disadvantaged of the AHA; the AHA advisory panel on Malpractice; a joint task force with the American Society for Hospital Attorneys; and a committee of the National Academy of Sciences on Research in V.A. hospitals. Society members have also participated in AHA-sponsored institutes on hospital law and seminars on risk management. The Society assisted in the development of a film on the patient representative's role in hospital risk management. At the American Health Congress in 1974, a slide/sound presentation "Let's Keep in Touch" that had been developed with the assistance of the Society Committee on Professional Development gave health professionals a view of the patient representative role. Other presentations were "Will the Real Patient Representative Please Stand Up!" "Health Care with Dignity: The Patient Representative Concept," "The Role of Volunteers in Patient Representative Programs," "Humanizing the Hospital."

At the local level, regional and state meetings have heard patient representatives describe their roles and functions in humanizing hospital care, in support of patients' rights, and as catalysts for systems change in health care institutions.

A Look Toward the Future

The objectives set forth at the beginning of the organization remain the focus of Society activities: presenting educational programs and activities to develop and strengthen programs, providing a medium of exchange and information among members, and disseminating information about patient representation to health care institutions and agencies.

The current climate points toward continued growth in numbers, size, and scope of programs. Many programs now include patients served in ambulatory care departments both within institutions, in free standing clinics, and in health maintenance organizations. At least one patient representative is employed in 1,425 AHA member institutions. Despite the push for economy, the latest AHA annual survey indicates that patient representation is one of the three areas of biggest spending growth in the hospital field. This increase is due to the continued demand for humanizing and personalizing the health care system, the perceived need for an interface between the consumer and the provider of health care, the breakdown in the doctor/patient relationship, and the publicity afforded the *Patients' Bill of Rights*. Other reasons for the growth are the increasing cost of health care that makes for greater demands by the consumer, the recommendation by some state legislatures, insurance underwriters, and the American Bar Association that patient representatives serve as the patient grievance mechanisms, and the demands of the "Freedom of Information" regulations in government facilities.

The early issue of placement of the program in the institution has been largely resolved. Most representatives report to top or second-level administration; some are assistant or associate directors of their institutions, as well as heads of the patient representative department, and participate as active members of management committees. This placement is advantageous in many respects but may be a deterrent in others. Representatives must be able to distance themselves from the problems and priorities of management, and focus attention on patient needs. This distancing is essential to the change agent role and may be *difficult* to maintain if patient representatives are an integral component of the administrative group.

Just as the early acceptance of this new field into the organization of the AHA was seen by some people as a means of preventing confrontation from outside the health care organizations, so acceptance as part of the management team may be an attempt (conscious or unconscious) at cooptation of patient representatives by the system. An example of this concern is surfacing as some representatives become active members of hospital "risk management" teams. Patient representative responsibilities, such as improving the climate of the institution and opening interdepartmental communications, make a direct impact on risk management efforts. However, if representatives assume the task of investigating incidents for management and negotiating directly with patients on behalf of the institution in possible malpractice or negligence suits, the advocacy role may become secondary and the focus of the occupation as it is now defined may shift.

There is still public concern about the effectiveness for the patient of an advocate appointed by and responsible to the health care institution. The Society points out that as members of hospital staffs, representatives can more readily negotiate for improved service for individual patients, investigate problems, and deal with them as they occur rather than after the fact. By serving as a central bank for registration of problems and concerns, representatives can accumulate data to pinpoint needed system change. However, confrontation by organized groups outside the institution may be more effective in the push toward major reforms in the health delivery system.[5]

Two of the role models on which patient representation is based are the Ombudsman concept, which is totally professional, and the Citizens Advice Bureau, wholly nonprofessional.[6,7] It is essential that patient representatives keep these two divergent roles in balance, staying close to patients, humanizing and individualizing health care, as well as advocating for change. The Society does not have "professionalism" of the field as a stated goal at present. Some members feel that becoming "professional" would create a barrier between them and those they serve. They agree with Dr. Paul Cornely who warned that the Society "should shy away from the models of medicine, nursing, and hospital administration." He stated that entry "should be an open one in which degrees and paper qualifications would not be the role standard."[8] Other members refer to themselves as professionals. The better educated and more sophisticated members the Society is now attracting may be interested in pushing toward professionalization. The government may also contribute to this move if educational and other job qualifications are established for staff of mandated patient grievance mechanisms. If it becomes advantageous to establish the field as a "profession" some of the necessary steps have already been taken.

Patient representation continues to grow and is beginning to be viewed as an integral component of health care. The Society has played a major supporting role in this growth.

References

1. Society of Patient Representatives of the AHA. *Essentials of Patient Representative Programs in Hospitals.* Chicago, American Hospital Association, 1978, p. 4.

2. Evelyn M. McNamara and Arline B. Sax. "Questions/Answers, Hospital Social Workers and Patient Representatives." *Hospitals* 48:9:14, May 1, 1974.

3. Society of Patient Representatives of the AHA. *Proposed Guidelines for a Patient Grievance Mechanism Approved by the Board of Directors.* Chicago, American Hospital Association, June 16–17, 1977.

4. Society of Patient Representatives of the AHA. *Guidelines for the Use of Volunteers in Patient Representative Programs in Health Care Institutions Approved by the Board of Directors.* Chicago, American Hospital Association, June 16–17, 1977.

5. Ruth Ravich and Helen Rehr. "Ombudsman Program Provides Feedback." *Hospitals* 48:18:63–67, September 16, 1974.

6. H.S. Reuss, and S.V. Anderson. "The ombudsman: tribune of the people." *Annals of American Academy of Politics and Social Science* 363:44–51, January 1966.

7. Alfred J. Kahn. *Neighborhood Information Centers: A Study and Some Proposals.* New York, Columbia University School of Social Work, 1966, pp. 33–35.

8. Paul B. Cornely. Address delivered at the Annual Meeting of the Society of Patient Representatives, A.H.A., Denver, Colorado, October 12, 1973.

Part IV

In the Patient's Interest: A Past and Future Look

Chapter IX

Dilemmas, Conclusions and Recommendations

HELEN REHR AND MILDRED D. MAILICK

A complex set of dynamics affects the health care system in its delivery of care to the public, the response of the public in general, and as individuals in that multidimensional, pluralistic system of services. This chapter deals with what the organized system can do through responsible providers at the service level and planners at the policy levels, what an individual can do in his own behalf, and what groups can do on behalf of the public. It does not deal with medical wrongdoing, malpractice, or malfeasance. Those problems belong in systems that permit legal redress in which both parties can be represented and situations adjudicated. While it is true that service delivery problems that can affect more than the individual complainant may be uncovered through medico-legal suits, these are after the-fact situations.

This chapter will deal with those problems of both human and organizational etiology and offer some problem resolution approaches to those who need and use the services, those who provide them, and those who are responsible for policy-making decisions for the services. Many studies have been done and a great deal has been written in relation to medical institutions as complex organizations and how organizations can achieve change. That literature will be drawn upon only as it pertains to affecting human behavior, the quality of relationships, and the way services are delivered "in the patient's interest."

Health and medical care have become a national preoccupation. Yet the medical care system is so incredibly complex that it is difficult to understand its intricacies and to disentangle and clarify its implications for the consumer. Except in relation to the patient role, insufficient attention has been devoted in the literature to understanding the patient as an active member of the health care system. The patient traditionally has been considered as the "object to be worked on," as a person from whom

"compliance" is to be elicited, or as someone who is passive or merely
reacting to other forces. The patients' interests in the medical care system
are quite evident: to be cured or to be returned to the highest possible
degree of functioning, quickly, painlessly, and at the least cost. In a large
measure, these interests were considered to be coterminous with those of
the medical care system as a whole, and therefore it was assumed that
innovation and technological improvements in the medical care system
served the patient as well.

Patients As Consumers

Only recently have we begun to consider patients more realistically
as consumers of medical services and to understand that they may indeed
have interests and perspectives that are divergent or even antithetical to
those who control the health care system. The definition of "who" the
patients are is also being reconsidered as the scope of attention is broadened to include individuals who are trying to gain access to the system and
those needing health care services but not attempting to receive them.

Considering the health care system from the point of view of patients
brings into focus a number of issues and problems that have been analyzed
before in other contexts, but which take on a new aspect when viewed from
the vantage point of patients. Thus, the responses of patients to problems
in the organization of the health care system throw a somewhat different
cast on their assessment. Similarly, considering how patients locate, gain
access, cope with, and evaluate medical care suggests a variety of ways in
which services to individuals may need improvement or reorganization.

One major dilemma for consumers as active participants in the health
encounter is that they lack expert knowledge about the services they need.
Another is that often they enter the health care arena at a time of personal
uncertainty and crisis, threatened by fear of illness and consequent loss
and personal jeopardy. These and other factors place patients in a position
of vulnerability and powerlessness in relation to health care providers.
Comparatively few mechanisms have been instituted to rectify this imbal-
ance.

Information

Information becomes the single most significant component among
the many that serve the orderly pursuit of problem solving. Information
is essential, but it must be in the hands of those who can work in relation
to its meaningfulness. People who have access to information can be in a
position of influence which can be used to serve their own interests. This
influence can be positive in relation to seeking beneficial change or nega-

tive by withholding, selecting, or using information to impede benefits.

Information, in order to be put to use, needs to be addressed in an organized and systematic way. The problem needs to be perceived, recognized, and openly acknowledged. Those who are involved with the problem, either in creating the difficulty or as recipients of it, need to acknowledge its existence before they can or will act on it. Individuals who are involved must also want to do something about it; that is, be motivated to examine it for its meaningfulness to all parties. Having identified the problem, a person must learn enough about it to understand why it happens. This takes collecting information through any means available, but two key means are observing and listening. Someone does need to assume responsibility for leading this process. Once gathered, the information needs to be sorted, analyzed, and evaluated. Understanding the problem in human factor terms, whether an individual consumer or the organizational providers, is critical. Who will be motivated to consider change and deal with the problem, who will not, and who may impede the process, need to be known.

Change has to be understood in the interest of those involved, and to be perceived as in their benefit before any alteration can occur. Not infrequently, this becomes a key process—working with the parties involved—in heightening awareness and in creating a desire for change. Whether consumer or provider, each must perceive the problem, wish for change, become invested in its implementation, periodically review the outcome, test for results, and report back to a source so as to justify the problem-to-problem-resolution process.

When problems exist between providers and consumers, for whatever reason, they must be brought out in the open so they can be viewed and dealt with. Problem solving requires information, data, knowledge, interpretation, and understanding. Out of this process alternatives as resolutions can be projected. When the problem involves more than one individual, which patient and provider encounters invariably do, then conscious awareness of the internal and external factors which impinge on it is required. Informal and formal channels of communication within the given health care system may well be involved, as well as interpersonal relationships between patients and significant others.

Consumer Responsibility for Health

It has been suggested by some health experts that the health status of consumers is determined by the responsibility they assume for their way of daily living. This means what they eat, what they do and how they do it, and the environment in which they live are believed as important to health maintenance as medical technology. These experts note that almost all of us are born healthy and become sick as a result of two critical factors: our personal misbehavior and environmental impacts. The responsibility for prevention of illness, that is, health maintenance, is placed on intelligent life-styles—what each individual does or does not do for himself. These experts call for a "self-help" approach and suggest that a "do unto thyself" care may be more efficacious than that of the physician. Oddly enough this point of view comes both from those who defend medicine and those who criticize it.[1-5] There are voices which suggest the medical care system is stretched beyond its potential; it is overcommitted and the expectations of the public are beyond what medicine can produce and therefore medicine should not be blamed. Some of these apologists go so far as to "blame" individuals for their failure to be well largely because they are motivated toward lifestyles that can be destructive or unresponsive to medical advice.

Other critics suggest that American medicine has over-medicalized the public in the "overprescription" of drugs and in the promise of technical aids. The belief promulgated is that medicine has contributed to human dependency and that individuals no longer know how to "care" for themselves. Medicine is responsible for a "sick" orientation of the public rather than an approach emphasizing wellness. This dependency accounts for the vast majority of all patients making office visits for symptoms arising essentially out of psychological stress and minor physical symptoms.[6,7] They are described as the "worried well," needing counseling, support, and comforting. It is acknowledged that little is available in the way of medical technology (other than the ready access to drugs) to deal with these "functional" distresses.[8] The recommendations of those who support demedicalization call for a different responsibility from the individual and a different allocation of scarce resources, less to medical programs and more to affect environmental health, including housing, sanitation, and working conditions.

These dichotomies in professional opinions put the issues into the medical, health, and consumer marketplaces. Criticisms of the medical care system or the public's behavior do not in any way lessen the public's demand for medical services. The concerns that we face deal with sound utilization by individuals, the development of motivation, and self-investment.

The perception of illness by individuals is a key factor in how they use the medical system. People who are sick and feel sick, who go through various steps from perceived need to utilization, have found the entryways to care. They then are dependent on what the medical care system offers them. Another group of people are "well" or "not sick," but feel sick, identify a problem, and reach a medical service. This large population may require other types of services after their symptoms have been medically screened. It is most likely that many patients who go to doctors' offices will obtain less expert care than if they had been referred to specialists in rehabilitation or in counseling; to programs that provide specific help—economic, housing, educational—; to such self-help groups as Weight Watchers, Alcoholics Anonymous or Gamblers Anonymous; or to those groups that are disease-specific, such as the American Cancer Society and the American Lung Association. The program a person reaches and the timing of that encounter may be key factors in the nature, quality, and meaningfulness of the service.

A third group, those who are sick but have not perceived a need for care are "at risk" and must be found. Many of these people will have conditions that are self-limiting. However, to ignore individuals whose illnesses are not contained is to place a severe burden on them, on the general population, and on services. Those who do not perceive the need for care have a general tendency to seek care late, when symptoms may already be irreversible. "Outreach" programs are needed to uncover individuals in need. These programs are most successful when they are localized, carried out in partnership between lay community people and specialists. The most important factor is not only screening and casefinding but the follow-through to help motivate individuals to use available services.

Health Education

There is always a need to inform individuals with disease about their illnesses and how to cope with them. Information is most valuable when it comes with programs which help individuals learn what they must do in their own interest, help them draw on their internal resources and become informed about available external assistance programs. Motivating individuals in their own behalf is the sine qua non in being able to help. The responsibility lies initially with individuals, but they need the support of the primary caretakers.

Physicians need to develop the "know-how" of helping people follow advice. Counseling services using professionally trained health social workers have demonstrated their helpfulness in developing motivation in individuals. In addition, social workers have been a resource to other practitioners for information about how to deal with patients and give information about available resources to meet patients' needs. When to make referrals to other experts or to specialized groups needs to be part of the education of all health care professionals. Learning to deal with noncompliant and dropout patients, learning how to reach out to those in need, and helping make each individual a better consumer of services should be part of the educational content as well.

There is a side of health education that deals with prevention of major difficulties. In schools and in clinics there are a great number of information programs which deal with the impact of overweight, smoking, and drug and alcohol abuses. These are largely local endeavors offering information with a premise that being informed leads to incentive to action. The program educators sometimes do not take into account all the social forces which serve to act as pressures on individuals. The educators assume that logic and understanding of self-destructive action will lead to corrective behaviors. If logic is not introduced, then fear is frequently used as a communication tool. There is evidence that neither incentive, punishment, nor prohibition tends to be effective in securing changed behavior.

Health education on a large scale through the media addresses a mixed population. There is indication that the broad sweep approach is not generally effective since it does not allow for differentiating the listening audience. A mosaic of approaches appears essential, and needs to identify the target population, the objectives, and the strategy of prevention. This calls for constant study of programs, learning more about those needing help, separating specific types into homogeneous groups, setting goals which are realistic, and, within time limits, using a wide range of methods in combination.

Studies are needed which can predict persons "at risk" and even when a crisis is likely to occur. A range of trial and error methods are also needed to reach such people.

One major concern is for the individual who reaches a medical care service but does not follow advice. An individual-client or patient is in noncompliance with medical recommendations and advice when he (a) accepts treatment and does not follow recommendations, (b) drops out of care, or (c) remains in treatment, but only partially follows the recommendations.

There is no question that all individuals who visit physicians need to take some action themselves in order to deal with the symptoms they present. The degree and the type of responsibility for such personal action varies greatly due to a wide range and combination of internal and external factors. Little seems to be known about the relationship of "following advice" to generating health maintenance. However, there is evidence that "following advice" in a range of conditions can be helpful in reducing symptoms, discomfort, disability, and even, perhaps, in avoiding death.[9] The logical assumption that most of us accept is that "following medical advice" should mean improvement of the sick state. Yet a large number of people fail to comply with recommendations. In general, the pattern of compliance which has evolved from many studies reveals that one-third do follow advice, one-third sometimes do, and one-third seldom or never do. The interesting consistent finding from studies is that physicians believe their patients are responding to their recommendations when in fact as many as one-half may not be complying. What has been demonstrated is that noncomplying patients very often do not reveal to their physicians that they are not following advice, especially if they are not asked.

Why don't people follow advice? Unfortunately, there are no clear-cut reasons. Neither age, sex, educational or income status, nor racial background is a critical deterrent to following advice. In examining personality traits there are only inconsistent and inconclusive findings about who will comply. Common sense suggests that if people understand their illnesses, how to deal with them, and why and how they can be controlled, they will most likely follow the advice. However, studies indicate that being informed does not make it happen. What seems to be helpful in getting individuals to respond to what they need to do is a combination of factors which together enhance motivation:

The physician's continuing expression of interest, even exhortation
A simplified regimen, of either dietary or personal habits, compatible with usual life style
The family's support of the regimen, even to "joining in" or for willing supervision
Trade-offs which may mean medication versus giving up salt or smoking, or setting limited goals over staggered time periods
Explicit and written instructions, tested for understanding and often repeated
Developing associations to effect the recall for doing what has to be done, and making it as routine and simple as possible
A short-term beneficial outcome so a sense of reward and achievement can be gained, then add next steps.

These reflect a few methods that take into consideration a partnership between patient and practitioner. The problem needs to be defined with clarity. Practitioners cannot expect patients to "do it" on their own. While there are those who say it is the individual patient who must assume responsibility, there is every indication that the patient will need to be helped. Their feelings, anxieties, and fears may get in the way. In addition to the physician-patient partnership, the family must be recognized as a major aid in whether what is needed by the patient will be supported. It is difficult to conduct a lone and single uphill course in a household of others. The environment in which one lives is also critical. Suggested behavioral changes must be feasible and compatible with the way one lives and the opportunities available and possible. While in the final analysis the individuals need to act in their own interests, they tend to do so more readily in a supportive and understanding atmosphere.

Access to Care

Other types of information have potential from the patient's point of view. Individuals need to learn skills in deciding whether, how, and when to enter the health care system. Comprehensive, community-based, health-oriented information and referral programs could play a role in improving the capacity of individuals to make such decisions, but they are not widely available. Some information and referral services concerned with health problems do exist, but they are usually devoted to serving the needs of single illness patient groups, such as diabetics; age categories, such as the elderly; or subject area, such as sex information. The major problem here is that these services are highly specialized. They stand as gatekeepers to resources, but potential patients must fit into a category in order to be eligible. Optimally, community-based services should be less specialized and serve a broader patient population. They should define their clients not only as those who cross their threshold asking for service, but also those who may require active outreach across cultural, economic, and psychological barriers.

Most access to medical care services is controlled directly by health care providers. In the absence of a universal health care system in which services are available to all, attention must be paid to the constriction of access to essential services for certain groups. Physicians are not coerced into accepting patients whom they do not wish to serve (Medicaid, chronically ill, elderly, minorities), to practice in geographical regions that are unattractive to them (urban ghettos, rural areas), or to develop specific medical competencies (general or family medicine, public health). When private practitioners do not provide care, institutional services (emergency rooms, hospital clinics, or government health services) may offer access. This leads to a two-tier system of medical care and with it major concerns about inequities in the quality of service. There are just the beginnings of government incentive programs to redistribute medical service, but this holds only marginal potential for dealing with some of the problems of access.

Hospital clinics and emergency rooms serve a large group of people, especially the urban poor who cannot or do not seek out private physicians. These institutions also have gatekeepers who screen in and out certain categories of patients. Hospitals with strong research and teaching interests may select patients for admission to services with priority given to those interests. Other clinics have financial barriers. They may accept only those who are covered by Medicaid, thus excluding the near poor who may find it especially difficult to get service anywhere. Inpatient services are also constricted. Many voluntary hospitals require proof of some form of medical insurance coverage from a patient or a large cash deposit prior to admission, except in cases of emergency.

Organized Consumers

Consumerism in the health care arena has been slow in developing. Inpatient care imposes a series of constraints upon patients and families that mitigates against the expression of consumer demand. In addition to medical care being highly individual in nature, patients are, or feel themselves to be, vulnerable by virtue of their dependence upon the hospital staff for maintenance of their body integrity and even for survival. Often physically uncomfortable or debilitated, they are away from their natural context and, at least for a period of time, captives in a closed institution. Their dominant responses are usually to adapt, to acquiesce, and to be "good" patients. They have little motivation to form coalitions with other patients with whom they see nothing in common except shared and transitory occupancy in the same institution.

Even if patients wish to find other patients with similar concerns about quality of care, they are obstructed by their inability to circumvent the barriers of the confidentiality of records. The institution itself cannot help them. It cannot share records or select patients who might be willing to be involved without getting prior and informed consent.

The quandary of hospitalized patients has been the subject of considerable attention, and hospitals have responded to recommendations of sociologists and psychiatrists with certain innovations. Efforts to improve the milieu for patients have led to better coordination of care, patient group meetings, and other innovations to reduce the many problems that patients may encounter. Also, community-based special interest groups, such as Reach for Recovery, have been allowed into hospitals and, in cooperation with staff members, have affected the care of certain patient groups.

Outpatient care has not received as much attention. While hospitals have made changes in terms of scheduling patients and developing triage mechanisms for emergency rooms, many problems remain. Clinic patients are likely to be more homogeneous in socioeconomic and ethnic status, and therefore have a greater potential for being politicized. Yet, they have remained vulnerable in most cases, unable to exercise pressure on their own behalf.

There is no general nationally organized consumer health movement that provides a countervailing force to the powerful organizations of the health care providers: the American Medical Association and the American Hospital Association. The national health advocacy organizations that exist are more interested in legislation and policy change than in resolving problems for individual patients. Most of them have a special interest in a single illness (diabetes, heart disease, cancer) and some of them are provider dominated. Many have major fund-raising functions, support research and specialized treatment, and lobby for legislation favorable to their constituencies. They compete with each other at national and local levels for funds and other resources, thus creating a fragmented and, at times, chaotic scene.

Organizations that do engage in case advocacy do not serve the general patient population. Veterans groups are most notable for their advocacy for their own constituency, not only at a legislative and policy level, but in support of individual members. They have considerable political power and can enlist intervention by congressmen and other officials in health matters, but only on behalf of their own members. Self-help groups, organized by patients themselves to deal with some of the gaps in service that they experience, are usually concerned with a single or related group of diseases or disabilities. Increasing numbers of these groups have been established in the past decade, mostly at a local level. They serve an important function, providing each other with information, emotional support, and skills for coping with their illness or disability. They encourage patients to advocate for themselves and have shown a potential for becoming a vital force in pursuing advocacy more actively. They have already been successful in using existing legislation to ensure the rights of their patient groups to fair employment practices and equity in insurance regulations.

All of these organizations provide a patchwork of services, both in relation to access and ongoing care, but none is open to an individual who does not fit into a specific category. Patients who do not know how to negotiate the health system or who cannot be identified with one category or another are at a disadvantage in gaining access to appropriate service. Community boards of voluntary and public hospitals and local Health Systems Agencies, which by law have more than 50 percent consumer representation, are potential sources of this kind of advocacy. They could provide a comprehensive approach on a communitywide basis, have a high degree of accessibility and visibility, and would be close enough to the major health institutions in the community to influence them on patients' behalf. Thus far, they have not taken on this role to any significant extent.

In addition to advocacy for the individual case, consumers in an organized movement must find ways to make an impact on the political process and regional and institutional planning. A partnership of patient consumers, professionals, and politicians needs to develop. If planning and policy-making are left to the influence of providers alone, we can expect no major change in the system. Codetermination means that all parties affected by the health care delivery system have equal responsibility in the process. The problems consumer movements face are many. Finding active, open-minded consumers and holding them in the movement has been difficult. Most prevalent is the rising influence of special interest groups, lay or provider, which have assumed leadership in the political process. In any event, what is essential for consumer-participants is ready availability of sound information and data. Being informed is the first essential step in order to put information to use.

Consumer groups need to develop and strengthen their voices in determining policy and program. They need to be heard where it counts.

This will call for organized efforts at the local and regional levels where they should:

Participate at the delivery of care level through membership on hospital, health maintenance, and other organizational advisory boards

Participate at the regional planning levels to include community boards, health system agency boards (HSA), professional standard review boards (PSRO), and other such groups

Develop and participate in programs for sharing information with the public on types of care, professionals and their services, costs and availability and how to use them to allow for informed choice and expectations

Develop and participate in community programs of sound case-finding and referral to needed services

Develop and participate in grievance and complaint machinery within institutions and in regional set-ups

Identify regional concerns and priorities, and participate in making them known

Develop up-front ways to talk with professionals, as individuals and to their professional organizations in order to help them understand individual patient needs

Develop mechanisms to hold institutions responsible for their programs and the way they deliver care through patients' rights information, patient representatives, ombudsmen, and consumer representation

Participate in organized professional accountability machinery, and develop the means to secure accountability to the consumer as well

Develop the means to become knowledgeable about illnesses, diseases, and disabilities along with their etiologies, treatments, impact, and the unknowns

Participate in the development of new health workers as links between providers and consumers

Work with a wide range of organizations dealing with medical and health issues: legal, women's movement, and disease-specific organizations

Become active in the political arena in order to affect choices, equity in availability, accessibility, and distribution.

Information gathering will help to determine what is missing, what is available, what is needed, the priorities, the resources, and further required information for questions that arise. The consumer group will need to secure whatever it requires from available sources. No matter what the group, it must have the resources to analyze and interpret the information it receives. The route to putting information to use for consumers is through organized efforts.

Satisfaction with care is a criterion that consumers can use. It may not be an indicator that "good" care has been delivered, nor does it mean that people who are "satisfied" necessarily "follow advice." What is known is that if there is dissatisfaction there may be problems in regard to using service, following through on advice, as well as in the nature of the provider-patient relationship. Many "satisfaction" studies are recognized to have flaws. However, they do offer an expression of attitudes and reactions from the consumer about the services received. These become important in addressing the difficulties and obstacles that exist in the social and organizational structure of the medical care system. Satisfaction and case studies should be conducted by consumer as well as provider groups as one way of securing consumers' responses to care.

Quality Assurance

A major concern for most patients is the quality of care that is received. There are two aspects of quality of medical services that are important to consumers. One relates to assessment of the technical excellence of the medical care, and the other to how the services are provided. These two aspects of quality are interdependent. While technical excellence rests on the establishment of standards of medical care and assessment of whether, in each individual case, those standards have been met, service delivery focuses on the quality of the interaction between the health care providers and patients in the interests of maximizing benefits to patients and minimizing the risks.

The consumer usually has very little part in the process of evaluating technical excellence. These judgments are almost always controlled by professionals. Traditionally, patients have been considered to have insufficient expertise to judge technical aspects of care and too emotionally involved to be objective. Even when a patient initiates an evaluation of the quality of care, it is another physician who is asked for a consultation or "second opinion." In cases of malpractice, a physician again is the one who acts as an expert witness on the issue of whether the quality of medical care meets established standards.

Recourse to the courts as a means of redress of grievance for negligence was established in England as early as the 14th Century, but until recently physicians protected the interests of their professional colleagues more assiduously than those of the consumers. Perhaps because the balance in malpractice cases is changing in favor of the consumer, the need for some intermediate means of redress of grievance and resolution of problems is being viewed with greater interest by the providers of health and medical care and by government agencies.

As long as medical care is provided in hospitals or other institutions peer review is likely to remain the principal form of quality control. Not only are patients' concerns rarely represented in these reviews, but they have had little or no access to their results. Physicians have traditionally protected their personal, professional, institutional, and class interests in all but the most flagrant cases of poor quality of care. The 1972 Amendments to the Social Security Act directed the establishment of Professional Standards Review Organizations (PSROs) in order to monitor hospital and nursing home care. While the implications of this legislation are not yet clear for physicians, other health care professionals, or the consumer, there is justifiable concern that physicians will continue to be governed by vested interests rather than by conscientious implementation of the mandate of the legislation. Even under circumstances where PSRO standards are scrupulously applied, the problem of availability of results of reviews to patients remains.

This oligarchy of power by physicians in judging the quality of medical care has been loosened to a limited extent in a small number of hospitals by the addition of a legal and consumer representative to the team involved in responding to complaints involving possible malpractice suits. Called "risk managers," these individuals investigate complaints and try to work out settlements that prevent patients from going to court. While this sometimes may be in patients' interests because it offers them an opportunity to settle grievances promptly without court procedures, it is clear that the risk managers are functionaries of the hospital and serve the patients ultimately only in the interests of the hospital's goals. When there is a clash between them, patients are well advised to have representation from outside the hospital. The elderly, the poor, and minority groups who are generally underserved by the legal profession are at a disadvantage and need more advocacy from community-based organizations than they receive.

It is interesting to note that the individual consumer of medical care services believes that the health system should be changed. Yet when asked, the vast majority do think good medical care can be obtained in this country. The major difficulties expressed are in the areas of cost, accessibility, and those areas which deal with interpersonal relationships between patient and physician. These latter concerns are with the quality of communication, understanding, friendliness, and responsiveness. Patients' concerns are for the human nature side of care and for the degree of time, thoroughness, and investment practitioners give.

Assessment of the quality of delivery of health care includes behaviors covering a range of professionals, paraprofessionals, and service workers, organizational arrangements, and activities broader than the evaluation of medical competence and technical skills. While assessment is complex, expert medical knowledge is not as crucial an issue. All individuals, although not unerringly correct in their judgments, have the potential for responding and evaluating in their own self-interest the quality of service of those who provide their care. It is, therefore, in relation to the assessment of service delivery that patients' responses are best heard.

Although the market mechanism is highly constricted in the area of health care, some patients can exercise choice and change physicians or clinics if the manner in which they are treated is considered unacceptable. However, for large segments of the population, such mobility is not feasible. In addition, it is in the interests of patients as well as providers that continuity of care be maintained. Therefore, mechanisms to resolve complaints about service delivery have increasingly been perceived as contributing to the quality of medical care.

In noninstitutional private practice settings, the expectation is that patients, when dissatisfied, will speak directly to providers. Despite the fact that this is perhaps the most open of the settings in which medical care is provided, patients often feel constrained and are reluctant to complain for fear of losing the favor of the physician. Almost no other mechanisms are available to resolve problems, as the few existing health advocacy organizations seldom take action against individual physicians except when flagrant abuses are involved. Similarly, lawyers are not eager to accept delivery of care cases which incur no demonstratable damage. Since there are no research data on how providers in solo or in small group practices are dealing with the problem, one can only conjecture about the number of individuals who may need medical care but who do not continue in treatment because they are reluctant or unable to resolve their problems with providers.

Medical care provided in institutions is both more complex and less responsive to individuals than it is in private practice settings, and issues of delivery of care are more complicated. The division of labor and stratification of specialties, level of technological sophistication, fragmentation and compartmentalization of services, and alienation of some service and professional workers all present difficulties from a patient's point of view. Institutional behavior is more difficult to assess and control. Inherent conflicts arise when highly autonomous professionals practice within the bureaucratic structure of a hospital or other health care institution.

The behavior of professionals is not subjected to the same degree of organizational control as service personnel. Professional decision making is essentially a personal responsibility, and it is guided by an internalized set of norms embodied in a code of ethics. Physicians and other professionals are monitored by peers and ultimately by the courts. Service workers derive their authority and make decisions in adherence with organizational rules and formal regulations. They are monitored and controlled by the supervisory process and surveillance. Since professional and service workers are interdependent, no one system of control is possible, and a conflict in authority may result in gaps in accountability. The patient whose needs are not being met may be caught in the confusion, not knowing how to lodge an appropriate complaint or to whom a complaint should be addressed.

Communication is intricate and often frustrating. In institutional settings formal feedback mechanisms about the delivery of care are more prevalent. These mechanisms are necessary for the institution as well as for patients. Hospitals have developed many administrative mechanisms for controlling and auditing the complex systems that contribute to their operation. However, only recently have some hospitals begun to perceive that information, not only *about* patients but *from* them can be useful. Patients are too often regarded as subjects of organizational manipulation. Their responses to care or the delivery of service are seldom elicited in any systematic way, except possibly in a post facto questionnaire. Yet, patients can contribute a crucial element to effective hospital management. When complaints are viewed as irritants and patients are viewed as persons who need to be controlled or placated, then the potential for putting information contained in their complaints to use is limited. However, if some dysfunction is viewed as inevitable in large, complex institutions and patients' complaints are seen as one possible indicator or tracer of the problems in the delivery of care that need attention, then they become a valuable source of information to the institution. A patient's view thus adds a dimension that cannot be provided by other component parts of the system. By itself, a patient's view is incomplete, but without it assessment of the quality of care is deficient.

Every department in the institution has responsibility for monitoring and evaluating the quality of its own service and, if it is large enough, it must have some formal mechanism for systematically doing so. However, each service has a tendency to cherish certain activities and work routines that are regarded as unalterably essential to their work. These are seen as immovable, and when complaints are evaluated each department tends to respond to them within this frame of reference. Patients' problems are apt to be explained away, considered unsolvable, or responsibility for them is projected onto another service. This avoids the necessity of the department to reexamine its own biases and search for novel solutions. This situation suggests that while a department may, and often does, devise a patient complaint channel within its own system, it is in a patient's interest to have another recourse that is interdepartmental, one that will view problems from a broader perspective. In addition, many problems reflected in a patient's complaint may implicate more than one department, and solutions must be worked out between them. As a result, an interdepartmental mechanism is needed, or one that provides access across departmental lines.

An institution can also identify areas of service that have a high risk for potential problems. Particularly in tertiary care hospitals, some services are inherently stressful for the staff, patients, and families. The hospital needs to be especially aware of these areas and must attempt to provide easily accessible channels through which complaints can be made and responded to. Hospitals serving vulnerable population groups may need to provide special mechanisms for feedback that bridge gaps in culture, class, age, or disability. These vulnerable groups may need to relate to someone who is indigenous to their own group, is highly visible and accessible, and helps patients to translate their complaints into a form or language that can be accepted into the hospital system.

Not all complaints and suggestions made by patients warrant a similar response. Very often, particularly in institutions, complaints are about problems that are unresolvable, either because they relate to medical or social situations of patients that cannot be relieved or altered, to government restrictions, or to the very complexity of the institution. Patients may sometimes use complaints about hospital care to express fear, pain, frustration, dependency, or anger that is related more to their physical or emotional state than it is to the problems complained about. These considerations must be taken into account. A referral to the social work department in many cases may be the most useful service. The crucial task is to avoid erring on the side of assuming that patients' complaints are unjustified because they are upset, confused, or ill, or on the side of taking all complaints at face value. This calls for decision making at a professional level of judgment.

Other complaints are quite specific to the unique situation of one or a very few patients. While these patients' problems need resolution, they are not usually indicators of system dysfunction or the need for organizational change. There is always the possibility that an infrequently occurring complaint might expose an important system problem. Depending on its severity and its potential consequences, the complaint can be responded to and resolved for the individual or can be acted upon for its implications for the system. However, when an aggregate of similar patient complaints and suggestions occurs, they should serve to point to trouble in the system and to suggest the need for administrative and professional review. The resolution of these complaints on an individual basis palliates the immediate problem for the patient and for the institution, but the latter has the responsibility, in the interests of prevention, to uncover and correct, if possible, the causes of the complaints. The expectation is not of a trouble-free system, but of one that is committed to the continuous review of problems as they surface from a variety of mechanisms of quality control.

In addition to receiving feedback from patients, the hospital has an interest in directing certain types of communication to patients, to reduce conflict between patients and itself. It is assumed that inherent in the relationship between them are some opposing interests that are partially amenable to resolution by the hospital through the provision of information. Patients in their own interest need information about the hospital, its expectations, rules, and the services it offers. Some of this is conveyed informally in terms of role expectations. The patient and family are expected to behave in certain culturally accepted ways, and are given cues by the staff about what is appropriate. This type of induced behavior is usually acceded to by patients as in their best interest and often proves to be so. However, sometimes the work style as well as the convenience and equanimity of the staff are considerations that are placed before the best interests of patients. Since the cues are subtle and patients are already vulnerable and at a disadvantage, it may be difficult for patients to respond to them or assert themselves, communicating their attitudes to those who are directly responsible for their comfort and care. An intermediary may be necessary. Also, when staff and patients do not share some of the language or cultural norms, informal cues may not be sufficient. Assistance may be required to bridge this gap.

Other hospital expectations and services are conveyed by written documents. These take the form of printed rules and descriptions of available services. Sometimes patients need help in translating these communications and in understanding them, either because they lack the language skills or physical capacity to understand the import of what is being conveyed in print. A system that provides this information in understandable form is in the interests of both patients and institution.

The *Patient's Bill of Rights,* adopted by many hospitals, is one form of conveying information to patients about what they can expect from the hospital and what their responsibilities are. While there are questions about the legal implications of the document as well as its efficacy, it usually impels an institution to designate someone whom patients can contact if they have complaints about those aspects of care referred to in it.

Patients also need information about their health, treatment being received, and alternatives to it. Not every patient can tolerate or use the same degree of involvement in understanding the treatments. Yet all patients should have some control over regulating the flow of information. The issue of a patient's right to know and informed consent involves ideological and ethical problems that have not been resolved. However, it is clear that the uncontested control of information by the medical establishment, which has been a factor in its power relations with consumers, is changing. Recent court decisions and government regulations about informed consent as well as the *Patient's Bill of Rights,* patient representative programs, and others are only a few manifestations of the direction of the change.

Thus a cluster of problems having to do with the relationship between the hospital and patients have become increasingly evident from patients' point of view. Many hospitals have established patient representative programs as one of the mechanisms for responding to a growing perception of patients' unmet needs. Almost all patient representative programs are involved in resolving complaints of one kind or another and in providing a liaison between the hospital and patients. The manner in which these functions are carried out and the kinds of complaints and information that are handled largely determine which of the three types of patient representative programs is developed—grievance, patient services, and hospitality programs. Distinctions having to do with goals and functions of each type of program are important as they implicate such issues as reduction of conflict, patient advocacy, data collection, system change, educational requirements, domain, and professional status.

Probably, no hospital employee can act as a advocate in its fullest sense within his or her own institution. At some point, an advisor or counselor based outside the hospital system is in a better position to represent the interests of patients. What is most helpful to the patient is to have both types of assistance; that is, a patient should have someone located inside the hospital who knows the workings of the system and can obtain services, remove obstacles, communicate information, reduce conflict, and resolve problems with prompt attention. In addition, a patient may need an advocate based outside the hospital who can respond to those complaints about institutional injustices that a patient representative or other staff members are unable or unwilling to entertain.

An important issue is whether patient representatives can be useful in a system whose values and interests are too far removed from those of patients. Some proprietary hospitals, and voluntary hospitals where research or teaching far outweigh service goals, might conceivably be institutions where this conflict could occur. Under such circumstances advocates, such as patient representatives who remain dependent on the administration of the institution for support, would neither resolve nor materially affect the problems of the patient. They might, in certain circumstances, be detrimental to the patient and even impede reform by reducing surface conflict. Patient representatives cannot be expected to effect institutional reform in a hostile setting, and there is considerable question about setting up such mechanisms when they give only the illusion of being in the interest of patients.

Consumer Influence on System Change

To involve patients in any systematic way as part of the change process, institutions must make sure that there are concrete structures for sensing their problems. Patient representative programs have varying potentials as sensing structures; they can tap different levels of problems in the system and have varying but always limited capacity to impel changes. Decision making and system change in even a small community hospital is a very complex process. It usually takes place slowly as a result of pressure from one or a coalition of interest groups within the hospital, strong pressure from the external environment either in the form of government regulations or funding requirements, a major breakthrough in technology, or an event dramatic enough to mobilize significant support. Patient complaints are seldom of sufficient influence by themselves to impel change except when combined with some other force. A patient's complaint can create pressure, tension, and heightened awareness about problems that may already or can easily be identified and supported by other segments of the hospital system.

Pressure from community-based ambulatory care patient groups can sometimes exert considerable influence. They have special potential for impelling system change in hospitals. In contrast to inpatients, they are only segmentally involved in the hospital system, and ordinarily are relatively powerless in influencing organizational change. However, when they represent a disaffected group, united by socioeconomic or ethnic identity, they become much more powerful. Large urban teaching hospitals are especially vulnerable to these groups. These hospitals assume a major responsibility for outpatient care of inner city populations. In addition, they often provide opportunities for service jobs for the poor and minority populations they also serve as patients. These institutions can become highly visible symbols of society's dysfunction, highlighting the economic and social chasm between providers and consumers and professionals and service workers. Civil rights groups and unions find these hospitals to be logical targets in their organizing efforts. Under circumstances of confrontation and the potential for violence, such outpatient groups can influence decision making, although permanent system change is more likely to occur if the groups are supported by other components or interest groups within the hospital. Relatively few patient representative programs function only in an outpatient setting, but those that do try to provide a mechanism that attempts to bridge the barriers between the institution and its patients, regulate and provide a channel for communication, and thus try to reduce the threat of confrontation.

Patient Representatives and System Change

Patient representative programs vary in the amount of authority vested in them to make recommendations or mandate change. Some grievance programs have the former function, but few have the latter. Without the power to make changes in the hospital system, some people question whether patient representatives can actively champion patients' rights. However, the authority to mandate change implies a degree of jurisdiction that would place patient representatives fairly high in the administrative hierarchy, with the attendant possibility of an overly close identification with institutional needs as opposed to patients' problems. The distinction between the role of a patient representative and that of a hospital administrator then becomes unclear. Patient representatives can best fulfill their function by helping an institution become aware of patient-perceived problems, documenting them, and, when appropriate, proposing workable solutions. Patient representatives most often act as catalysts, for as they identify gaps in service and other problems they focus the attention of the staff on the patients' perspectives. The responsibility for decision making and the implementation of change belongs with the professional, technical, and administrative staff.

Data collection and utilization are also dependent upon the purposes of the various types of patient representative programs. The greater the expectation that the program will contribute to the identification of and recommendations for resolution of problems, the more urgent the need for accurate record keeping and statistical reports. Grievance programs tend to have the most sophisticated and detailed records. When the program focus is on gaining access to services for the patient or the resolutions of patients' complaints rather than on the use of patient-based data for system change, the records kept are apt to be less detailed or elaborate.

Informal communication and personal contact are important and often necessary to motivate change, but unless they are supported by formal data and written communication, they seldom have the power to institutionalize change. This is especially so in institutions as complex as hospitals.

Professional Status of Patient Representatives

In the light of the programs' diversity of function, there are differences in the preparation and skills needed by patient representatives and in their level of professionalization. There seems to be agreement that certain personality characteristics, such as maturity, tact, judgment, sensitivity, tenacity, an ability to cope with stress, and a capacity to communicate effectively with a range of individuals, are important assets in patient representatives in order for them to function in any of the types of programs. However, there is less uniform agreement about the educational preparation and professional qualifications for employment appropriate to each type of program.

The functions of the grievance program require that patient representatives have the capacity to make discriminate judgments in evaluating patient complaints, intervening in patients' behalf, and communicating with appropriate staff members throughout the hospital. The essence of their activity is concerned with unique situations in which rules of operation established by the hospital either do not apply or create discomfort, hardship, or inequity for patients. Patient representatives, thus, must go beyond rule-governed behavior and draw on an internalized system of values and principles to guide their actions. This requires a professional orientation which is usually associated with educational preparation of at least and, more often beyond, the baccalaureate level. The other types of programs are not necessarily governed by the same requirements.

An analysis of the tasks of the hospitality program suggests that a much more limited degree of autonomy and responsibility is exercised. Here, individuals with less formal education who bring basic interpersonal skills, common sense, and intelligence are adequately prepared. The patient services programs, in which some forms of counseling and other direct services are provided, form a middle group. These programs have the most ambiguous functions and the level of education may vary with the complexity and responsibility of the activities performed by the patient representative in each hospital. In some cases, social work training may be required.

The issue of professionalization can be viewed in much the same way. It is the patient representatives in the grievance programs who have the most potential for moving toward professionalization. The other types of programs are not as dependent on professional status to attain their goals. Professionalism is a peculiarly sensitive issue in hospitals. The grievance patient representative lacking professional status might be handicapped in working with physicians, nurses, and other professional and technical members of the staff. Concern has been expressed by some people that education and professionalism will create sufficient social distance between patients and a patient representative to vitiate the usefulness of the program. This argument is based on the assumption that the higher education itself creates an unbridgeable social chasm between a patient and a representative. Research does not support this belief, nor does experience with indigenous workers in the poverty programs established in the 1960's. Rather, it was skills in system negotiation in conjunction with language skills in representatives that were ultimately the most useful attributes to minority and low income groups.

The patient representative group as a whole has moved to some degree towards professional status. Its main deterrent has been a lack of conceptual clarity about goals, functions, and activities. As long as the Society of Patient Representatives allows the present diversity of function without distinguishing between types of programs or developing differential standards for them, it will probably remain an amorphous occupation.

Occupational groups usually follow a series of well-defined and sequential steps in their progress toward professional status. They first establish a professional association with designated criteria for membership. This is followed by the adoption of a new name to point to their changing status. The development of a code of ethics is the next step. It provides a rationale to society for the professional group and imposes a set of norms on its members. Then follows a period in which the professional group, through its association, tries to get societal support for a limitation on the title of the occupation. At a later stage, there is an attempt to reserve the performance of certain activities to members of the profession. Concurrently, the professional society establishes and controls professional training facilities, thus regulating admission, socialization, and qualification of new recruits to the profession.[10]

Patient representatives have progressed beyond the first step in the process of professionalization. They formed an association in 1972 as an auxiliary of the American Hospital Association. (See Chapter 8) While its membership criteria are quite loosely drawn, not everyone who applies is accepted. Similarly, patient representatives have moved toward the adoption of one name, although many other titles are still accepted and used. The title currently used is overinclusive, encompassing a great range of individuals and activities. Further clarification of title is necessary. Until this has been accomplished, the association cannot meaningfully set standards or enforce norms for its membership. The patient representative group has not officially adopted a code of ethics. Some occupations try to increase their status by adopting a formal code of ethics before they have the power to enforce it. The patient representative group has opted for a statement of philosophy and goals which embodies a sense of service and responsibility for conduct toward patients. Realistically, the association is not strong enough to enforce compliance although the bylaws empower the board of directors of the society to expel members for cause. It does not have sufficient power to establish functions, qualifications, and norms of conduct or to intervene to protect its membership. It cannot challenge the hospitals, although by virtue of its relationship as an auxiliary of the American Hospital Association it has access to communication with the parent body. Under these circumstances, its membership will be more likely to owe allegiance and be oriented to the employing hospitals than to the national organization.

The problem of conceptual clarity of function has also created problems in establishing the domain of the patient representative group. The domain of a professional or occupational group is determined partly by the goals it sets for itself and the functions it performs in order to fulfill these goals. Each professional group asserts a series of functions that it actually performs and another series that constitutes its aspirations for future performance. The process of establishing a professional domain rests not only on a clear statement of both, but on the acceptance of the legitimacy of the claims by other elements in the system and society. It usually involves a process of conflict and negotiation. Patient representatives are at the beginning stage of this process of negotiation. The expectation is that over a period of time, in each of their hospitals and at the level of national associations, there will be further clarification of domain.

Social workers in particular have been concerned that patient representatives might usurp part of their domain. The two main functions in contest have been the advocacy functions of the grievance programs and the counseling and discharge functions of the patient services programs. In hospitals with traditional social work departments, in which the role is defined narrowly in terms of individual casework services, the advocacy function is not very highly valued or, in fact, claimed by many of the social workers. Even in hospitals where social work claims advocacy as part of its domain, this function may not be supported or even accepted by the administration or the professional staff. Without these sanctions, social workers, especially those providing direct service in collaboration with other professionals, find it difficult to advocate for patients. It creates problems in interprofessional relationships which endure long after an individual patient is no longer part of the hospital system. A patient representative who has no direct service role, is attached to no service area or unit, and is less involved in interdependent relationships in performing tasks may be less vulnerable when engaging in advocacy activities.

It is clearly within the line social worker's responsibility to deal with systems problems and advocate for patients when solutions to problems are available within the service area to which the social worker is assigned. Further responsibility depends on the professional conscience of each social worker, the milieu of the hospital, the guidelines and leadership of the social work department, and on the role that the patient representative might take.

Thus, the relationship between the social worker and the grievance type of patient representative is dependent upon how each views his or her functions and domain. The possibilities for an amicable division of labor or for overlap and conflict are both present. Individual circumstances in each hospital, in terms of the leadership qualities of the personnel involved as well as political and budget considerations, will affect how the division of responsibility takes place.

A possible optimal resolution of the domain issue might be to assign to the grievance patient representative program those problems of patients who encounter dysfunction in the hospital system that cannot be solved at the line level by the directly involved members of the staff or their immediate supervisors. The two principal functions of the patient representative program would be the gathering and channeling of data on patient care problems and the resolution of problems for patients for whom the existing procedures are not working effectively. The domain of the patient representative would be interdepartmental in nature, and thus allow for problem identification and resolution that would be more difficult for members of the staff who are assigned to a specific service.

The assignment of specific responsibility between the two programs —social work and patient representative—is likely to take place more or less informally on a case-by-case basis with the domains of each program as guidelines. Conflicts are likely to occur at points of overlap, but the potential also exists for a coalition of the two programs around important issues.

The patient services type of patient representative program poses quite different kinds of issues and problems from those of the grievance program. Patient services programs duplicate the core functions usually assigned to social work departments. Further, there are indications that these programs are more likely to be found in hospitals with poorly established and poorly professionalized social work departments with a narrow range of functions. The obvious but unanswered question is whether there is a reciprocal relationship between the two programs, that is, whether in some way the quality of the social work program created a situation that allowed a competitive program to be established. Patient representatives and social workers are at the beginning stages of the process of negotiation for domain. The expectation is that in time there will be further clarification of the role and function of each.

The issue of domain extends beyond the boundaries of hospitals. There are no clear or rigid lines of demarcation between the institutions and the external environment. Patient representatives, social workers, and others based within a hospital extend their services outside of its environs by helping patients to enter, receive appropriate service, and exit from the institution. However, they cannot deal with persons who do not enter its doorways or get drawn in by various special screening programs. It is here, at the interface between an institution and a community, that linkage between community-based information and referral systems and hospital-based programs must take place. This has the dual potential of ensuring entry to those who need care and avoiding or reducing inappropriate or wasteful use of valuable medical resources. It also serves to point up gaps in service for planners and legislators.

Conclusions

No matter how successful an institution or even an individual may be in the resolution of problems, there will always be new problems. An institution and its providers have a constant responsibility to assess what is being delivered and to diminish the obstacles that patients encounter. Wherever a system exists which deals with the interaction between a client and a provider, then a mechanism to deal with problems the parties may face needs to be created. The means to monitor, review, and correct fall within the service organization, either with those who deliver service or those who administer the service delivery. The means to deal with issues can be as broad as the perspectives of those in charge of service delivery and those involved in providing the service. The corrective machinery can be under the aegis of a single department covering its own emerging problems or under a centralized overall administrative mechanism; the latter has the advantage of being able to cross departmental lines. However, centralized mechanisms usually resolve one problem at a time and do not have the capability to involve departmental peer investment in the same way a single department's leadership can. What is required to deal with the melange of problems that complex (and even not so complex) organizations face is a mosaic of means.

Patient representative and social work programs are two methods by which medical institutions may deal with the problems patients face in the process of receiving care. It is apparent that patient representatives deal with the impediments in provider services that patients face. Social workers tend to deal more with factors that are concerned with the way patients utilize medical care. This involves interpersonal counseling and the motivation of patients and families to be responsive in their own interests. They are concerned with obstacles to care, and, in many instances, social workers do coordinate and link the multiple components of care for the individual. They tend to do less with institutional impediments.

Another key means to deal with the obstacles caused by hospital personnel is to reorient practitioners to be responsive to the individuality and human qualities of their patients. This calls for educational content for all health care professional students that covers concern not only for patients as individual consumers, but also for the quality of programs that fall under the social contract for the public good. This can be achieved only if educational institutions—medical, nursing, pharmacy, social work, hospital administration, and such—redirect their goals to safeguarding both the individual and public good.

Another obligation is vigilance within the medical setting about the quality of interrelationships between patients and the wide range of providers, both professional and paraprofessional. Vigilance requires information that covers review, assessment, and recommendations for change by those who are involved in delivering services. It is possible that the initiative for such periodic review can be department-based. This would mean that such departments as medicine, surgery, nursing, and social work would each have peer review programs to deal with professional practices and their own ombudsman to deal with all ancillary programs. The critical cue to successful periodic review is the participation by those involved. While patients must be vigilant in their own behalf, providers must maintain a service ideal and take measures to insure quality and equity.

References

1. John H. Knowles. "The Responsibility of the Individual." *Daedalus* 6:1:57–80, Winter, 1977.

2. Lewis Thomas. "On the Science and Technology of Medicine." *Daedalus* 6:1:35–46, Winter, 1977.

3. Renee C. Fox. "The Medicalization and Demedicalization of American Society." *Daedalus* 6:1:9–22, Winter, 1977.

4. Walsh McDermott. "Evaluating the Physician and His Technology." *Daedalus* 6:1:135–157, Winter, 1977.

5. Ivan Illich. *Medical Nemesis.* New York, Pantheon Books, 1972.

6. United States Department of Health, Education and Welfare, Public Health Service, Health Resources Administration. "The National Ambulatory Medical Care Survey: 1973 Summary," p. 22.

7. R. Anderson, et al, "Psychologically Related Illness and Health Services Utilization." *Medical Care* 15:5:42, May 1977, Supplement.

8. Lewis Thomas. *Op. cit.,* p. 42.

9. Robert K. Maddock, Jr. "Patient Cooperation in Taking Medicines." *Journal of the American Medical Association* 199:3:137–140, Jan. 16, 1967.

10. Herbert Caplow. "The Sequence of Professionalization." In *Professionalization,* Edited by Howard M. Vollmer and Donald Mills. Englewood Cliffs, Prentice-Hall, 1966, pp. 20–21.

DATE DUE

APR 18 1986			
May 8, 86			
May 28, 86			
June 18, 86			

GAYLORD PRINTED IN U.S.A.